"This is an important book! By means of its interdisciplinary approach, and at the intersection of translation and writing, it explores what it entails to be truly patient-centered. Scholars as well as practitioners within translation and health communication will benefit from topical insights on significant issues such as how to ensure comprehensibility, accommodate the target group, and support patients at an emotional level."

– Karen Korning Zethsen, Professor of Translation Studies at Aarhus University, Denmark

"A welcome work that explores the various dimensions of patient-centered communication and translation, increasingly at the heart of medical and paramedical practices. Comprehensive, well-documented and well structured, this must-have book for anyone designing or translating patient-facing documents will be useful to students and experienced professionals alike, as well as to teachers and researchers."

– Sylvie Vandaele, Full Professor, Université de Montréal, Canada

"I applaud the authors for their work on this long-awaited volume which explores different aspects of patient-centered translation, which should be essential reading for any student, educator or practitioner involved in this important field of community translation. Patients are the all-important end-users of health translation, and involving end-user perspectives in the final health translation product is crucial."

– Ineke Crezee, ONZM, Professor of Translation and Interpreting, Auckland University of Technology, Auckland, New Zealand

PATIENT-CENTRED TRANSLATION AND COMMUNICATION

In response to the growing importance and spread of patient-centred care, the need to empower patients and the trend towards democratising specialised knowledge in health care, this book puts patients centre stage and provides concepts, methods and learning materials to enhance effective communication with patients and relatives in health care settings.

Opening chapters establish the conceptual and methodological framework needed to understand patient-centredness, the crucial role of context and culture, the range of communicative situations and text genres involved and the diversity of modes, formats and media in which patient-centred translation and communication take place. Subsequent chapters raise awareness of the importance of carefully defining the target audience and producing understandable and empathetic messages and provide analytical tools for making decisions in these three key areas. The concluding chapter offers avenues for research in patient-centred translation and communication with the hope of bridging the gap between practice and research and advancing this growing field of inquiry.

Including activities, resources, summaries, further reading and pointers to further research in each chapter, this is the essential guide for all translators and interpreters, students and professionals working in this area of translation studies, health care and communication studies.

Vicent Montalt-Resurrecció is Full Professor in the Department of Translation and Communication Studies at the Universitat Jaume I, Spain. He is co-author of *Medical Translation Step by Step* (Routledge, 2007).

Isabel García-Izquierdo is Full Professor in the Department of Translation and Communication Studies at the Universitat Jaume I, Spain. She is author of *Divulgación médica y traducción. El género información para pacientes* (2009).

Ana Muñoz-Miquel is Professor in the Department of Translation and Communication Studies at the Universitat Jaume, Spain. She is the author of *La traducción médico-sanitaria: profesión y formación* (2023).

Translation Practices Explained

Series Editor: Kelly Washbourne

Translation Practices Explained is a series of coursebooks designed to help self-learners and students on translation and interpreting courses. Each volume focuses on a specific aspect of professional translation and interpreting practice, usually corresponding to courses available in translator – and interpreter-training institutions. The authors are practicing translators, interpreters, and/or translator or interpreter trainers. Although specialists, they explain their professional insights in a manner accessible to the wider learning public.

Each volume includes activities and exercises designed to help learners consolidate their knowledge, while updated reading lists and website addresses will also help individual learners gain further insight into the realities of professional practice.

Most recent titles in the series:

Legal Interpreting and Questioning Techniques Explained
Mira Kadrić, Monika Stempkowski and Ivana Havelak

Translating for Museums, Galleries and Heritage Sites
Robert Neather

Patient-Centred Translation and Communication
Vicent Montalt-Resurrecció, Isabel García-Izquierdo and Ana Muñoz-Miquel

For more information on any of these and other titles, or to order, please go to www.routledge.com/Translation-Practices-Explained/book-series/TPE

Additional resources for Translation and Interpreting Studies are available on the Routledge Translation Studies Portal: http://routledgetranslationstudiesportal.com/

PATIENT-CENTRED TRANSLATION AND COMMUNICATION

Vicent Montalt-Resurrecció,
Isabel García-Izquierdo and
Ana Muñoz-Miquel

Routledge
Taylor & Francis Group
LONDON AND NEW YORK

Designed cover image: SpicyTruffel

First published 2025
by Routledge
4 Park Square, Milton Park, Abingdon, Oxon OX14 4RN

and by Routledge
605 Third Avenue, New York, NY 10158

Routledge is an imprint of the Taylor & Francis Group, an informa business

British Library Cataloguing-in-Publication Data
A catalogue record for this book is available from the British Library

Names: Montalt i Resurrecció, Vicent, author. | García-Izquierdo, Isabel, author. | Muñoz-Miquel, Ana, author.
Title: Patient-centred translation and communication / Vicent Montalt-Resurrecció, Isabel García-Izquierdo and Ana Muñoz-Miquel.
Other titles: Translation practices explained. 1470-966X
Description: Abingdon, Oxon ; New York, NY : Routledge, 2025. | Series: Translation practices explained | Includes bibliographical references and index. |
Identifiers: LCCN 2024024028 (print) | LCCN 2024024029 (ebook) | ISBN 9780367281106 (hardback) | ISBN 9780367281120 (paperback) | ISBN 9780429299698 (ebook)
Subjects: MESH: Communication | Patient-Centered Care | Professional-Patient Relations | Culturally Competent Care—methods | Patient Education as Topic—methods | Translating
Classification: LCC R118 .M64 2025 (print) | LCC R118 (ebook) | NLM W 62 | DDC 610.1/4—dc23/eng/20240701
LC record available at https://lccn.loc.gov/2024024028
LC ebook record available at https://lccn.loc.gov/2024024029

ISBN: 978-0-367-28110-6 (hbk)
ISBN: 978-0-367-28112-0 (pbk)
ISBN: 978-0-429-29969-8 (ebk)

DOI: 10.4324/9780429299698

Typeset in Sabon
by Apex CoVantage, LLC

CONTENTS

Acknowledgements ix

Introduction 1

1 Understanding contexts in patient-centred communication 6

1.1 Understanding patient-centred communication 7
1.2 Exploring context 15
1.3 The concept of culture in patient-centred communication 19

2 Diversity of text genres for patients 27

2.1 The concept of genre 28
2.2 Introducing Olivia, our patient 32
2.3 Some current genres involving patients 33
2.4 Emerging genres involving patients 56

3 Exploring multiple modes, codes, formats and media 60

3.1 Approaching multimodality 61
3.2 Multimodality in the medical consultation 62
3.3 Accessibility and inclusivity 69
3.4 Expanding modes and formats 73

4 Analysing your target audience 79

4.1 Audiences and genres addressed to patients 80
4.2 Characterising the situation 83
4.3 Analysing the audience 87
4.4 Types of patients and their needs 92
4.5 Addressing your audience in a patient-centred way 98

5 Creating texts for patients: comprehensibility 100

5.1 Defining and characterising comprehesibility 101
5.2 Assessing comprehensibility 106
5.3 Some recommendations to improve comprehensibility 109

6 Creating texts for patients: empathy 115

6.1 What is empathy? 116
6.2 Empathy in oral communication 119
6.3 Empathy in written communication 126
6.4 Cultural variation in the expression of empathy 134

7 Starting research in patient-centred translation and communication 137

7.1 Research approaches, methods and tools in patient-centred translation and communication 138
7.2 Areas of interest 148
7.3 Some resources for research in patient-centred translation and communication 161

Glossary 164
Bibliography 170
Index 181

ACKNOWLEDGEMENTS

We would like to thank Kelly Washbourne, the editor of this series, for his invaluable guidance and support throughout the writing process. From the outset, Kelly responded to our drafts with a remarkable ability to embrace different perspectives. He understood the dialogue and intersections between translation, communication and patient-centred health care that inspired this book in the first place and encouraged a holistic approach to our work. Of course, any shortcomings that remain in this book are our responsibility.

We wish to acknowledge all we have learnt conducting research together as members of the Textual Genres for Translation (GENTT) research group at the Universitat Jaume I. For many years, we have had the privilege of conducting research in text genres for translation purposes, and more recently, in multilingual communication in clinical settings involving patients. As a research group, we have been fortunate to receive institutional support and public funding from various bodies, including the Spanish Ministry of Science and Innovation, the Regional Government of the Generalitat Valenciana and the Universitat Jaume I. We recognise that it is our duty and civic responsibility to reciprocate the investment society has made in us by contributing our knowledge and expertise for the betterment of society.

We are deeply indebted to the patients who shared their experiences of language and communication with us, particularly those from Carena, a patient association in Valencia, Spain. Their insights have profoundly enriched our understanding and inspired our work, making our scientific journey more meaningful and humane.

Finally, as co-authors of this book, we want to express our sincere gratitude to each other for the unwavering support and collaboration that drove the development of this manuscript. We appreciate the insights gained from sharing our experiences in research, teaching and professional roles to achieve our objective: to contribute to the understanding and improvement of translation and communication practices in patient-centred contexts. Despite the challenges, including those posed by the pandemic and personal hurdles, we are grateful for the teamwork that led to the completion of this work.

INTRODUCTION

> "The good physician treats the disease; the great physician treats the patient who has the disease."
>
> (William Osler)

Since *Medical Translation Step by Step. Learning by Drafting* was first published more than 15 years ago in this series, patient-centred communication and translation have become increasingly relevant. In the ever-evolving landscape of healthcare, the importance of both effective and empathetic communication cannot be overstated. The imperative to prioritise the patient's voice has turned into a central tenet of best practice in many healthcare systems. As the dynamics between healthcare professionals, health authorities, patients and their families continue to shift towards a patient-centred model of care, the role of language and communication as social and cultural determinants of health are increasingly coming to the fore.

Translation, conventionally understood as the conversion of text from one language to another, assumes a heightened significance within the realm of patient-centred care and communication in today's multilingual and multicultural societies. In addition to linguistic and conceptual accuracy, *patient-centred translation* (Montalt 2017) encompasses comprehensibility, cultural and emotional sensitivity, inclusivity, and the ability to bridge knowledge gaps effectively. How do we ensure that health information is not just translated but also culturally and cognitively adapted, fostering a deeper understanding and engagement from patients of diverse backgrounds?

Patient-centred Translation and Communication explores interdisciplinary spaces where patients, health, medicine, language, communication,

DOI: 10.4324/9780429299698-1

cognition, and translation are entangled and interact in ways that are relevant to a wide range of readers committed to improving the quality of healthcare communication in practice. As we navigate the diverse linguistic, cultural and informational landscapes that characterise contemporary healthcare in many countries, this volume is addressed to translator trainers, translation students and scholars, professional translators and interpreters as well as to health professionals, medical writers, medical students and trainers in the area of medical communication. It aims to provide a nuanced exploration of an emerging professional practice at the intersection of translation and writing within the paradigm of patient-centred care and communication, where little teaching and learning material is available to date.

Structure of the book

Chapter 1. Understanding contexts in patient-centred communication. In this chapter, we start from patient-centredness as a health paradigm that prioritises the needs and experiences of patients. It emphasises involving patients in their care, using their mother tongue, considering their values and preferences, and fostering a collaborative and respectful relationship with health professionals. Patient-centred care aims to ensure that healthcare decisions are made in the patient's best interests, taking into account their individual circumstances and goals. This approach recognises the importance of treating patients not just as recipients of medical care and information but as active participants in their own health and well-being through appropriate communication. In this paradigm, the importance of context and culture cannot be overemphasised, as they shape the way individuals perceive and interact with health information, influencing their understanding, decision-making and overall experience of the healthcare system. Patient-centred translation and writing that neglects these crucial factors can lead to miscommunication, reduced health literacy and poor patient outcomes.

Chapter 2. Diversity of text genres for patients. Patients are involved in myriad communicative situations, ranging from oral interactions with doctors in medical consultations to the expression of their personal experience of illness in written texts. All these communicative situations are articulated through a variety of text genres, many of which are typically written. In this chapter, we look at some of the most representative ones. Some are more standardised, such as the patient information leaflet, while others are less so, such as the patient narrative. Familiarity with their conventions and the way they are used in clinical situations is essential for communication practice in patient-centred environments. One of the main concerns of this chapter is that patients may be involved in a variety of communicative situations where different registers, styles and textual conventions are used. A fundamental premise of this chapter is that although the genres presented in this book are addressed to patients, not all of them are patient-centred and patient-friendly. In fact, there is much room for improvement to make them more accessible, understandable and empathetic, something that translators and writers need to consider.

Chapter 3. Exploring multiple modes, codes, formats and media. Multimodality in patient-centred translation and communication refers to the use of multiple modes or channels of communication, such as verbal, written, visual and digital, to convey health information and enable communication processes. In this chapter, we emphasise that the use of multimodality in patient-centred communication is crucial for several reasons. Patients have unique needs, preferences and levels of health literacy. Multimodal communication enables health professionals to tailor their messages to individual patients in the medical consultation and beyond, ensuring that information is presented in a way that is most accessible and meaningful to each person. Health literacy is a key determinant of patient understanding and engagement. Multimodal communication addresses different levels of health literacy. In addition, patients may have different abilities and limitations, such as hearing impairments, visual impairments or cognitive challenges. Multimodal communication takes these different abilities into account and ensures that information is accessible to all patients, regardless of their physical or cognitive limitations or circumstances. Health inequalities often result from communication challenges. Finally, the use of multimodality is consistent with the integration of digital technologies in healthcare. Patients increasingly engage with health information and communication through digital platforms, and a multimodal approach allows healthcare providers to adapt to changing technologies and to respond to patients' communication preferences.

Chapter 4. Analysing your target audience. Patients are not a single social group. There are many types of patients, and addressing each of them appropriately can be a challenge for communicators. Their strategies and choices will depend on the specific audiences they have in mind. In order to make texts more patient-centred, it is necessary to have a very clear and defined idea of the reader/recipient and what they will do with the information provided. In this chapter, we argue that depending on age, gender, disease and other factors, addressing diverse audiences in patient-centred communication is crucial to providing equitable and inclusive healthcare. Diverse audiences include people with different cultural backgrounds, languages, health literacy levels, abilities and preferences. For example, paediatric patients require communication approaches that are age-appropriate and take into account developmental stages. Geriatric patients may have specific communication needs related to age-related conditions, sensory impairments or cognitive changes. In this chapter, we also highlight that the patient's mother tongue is a fundamental element of patient-centred communication. Healthcare providers who prioritise and incorporate the patient's mother tongue into their communication practices contribute to a more inclusive, respectful and patient-centred healthcare experience.

Chapter 5. Creating texts for patients: comprehensibility. Much of the medical information with which patients are confronted originally comes from the biomedical domains in which health professionals specialise through their university education and clinical practice. Specialised registers permeate the clinical settings in which patients interact with health professionals. Although many genres are explicitly addressed to patients, comprehensibility remains a problematic area. In this chapter, we highlight that comprehensibility is highly relevant to patient-centred communication for several reasons. It is essential that patients fully understand their health conditions, treatment options and potential outcomes. When they have a clear understanding, they are better able to participate in shared decision-making processes and actively contribute to decisions about their care. In addition, patients are more likely to adhere to prescribed treatment plans when they understand the rationale behind them. Clear communication helps patients understand the importance of medications, lifestyle changes and follow-up appointments. Health inequalities are often caused by communication problems. Comprehensible communication is a critical factor in addressing these disparities by ensuring that health information is accessible and understandable to diverse populations, including those with varying levels of health literacy.

Chapter 6. Creating texts for patients: empathy. In this chapter, we focus on emotional aspects of patient-centred translation and communication, which are crucial to creating materials that resonate with individuals on a personal and empathetic level. Patient-centredness aims to communicate health information in a clear, compassionate and emotionally supportive way. Using an empathetic tone, personalisation strategies and compassionate language; addressing emotional concerns; acknowledging emotional impact; introducing positive reinforcement; being sensitive to cultural differences; respecting privacy and dignity and adapting texts to different emotional states are some of the ways to make texts and communication more patient-friendly. In this chapter, we will see that by integrating these emotional aspects into patient-centred translation and writing, healthcare providers as well as translators and writers can create materials that not only inform but also support patients on an emotional level, fostering a sense of connection, understanding, reassurance and empowerment.

Chapter 7. Starting research in patient-centred translation and communication. Research on patient-centred translation and communication is still in its infancy. In this final chapter, we briefly present a selection of research approaches, methods and tools that may be useful for investigating issues relevant to patient-centred translation and communication. We also present research areas, topics and questions derived from the previous chapters that focus on some of the most pressing needs, such as addressing different types of patients, comprehensibility, empathy or cultural issues. Examples of actual published research are provided to direct the reader to relevant articles that may be of interest in terms of conceptual and methodological ideas. Finally, we provide basic resources and tools that can help the budding researcher in the first steps of a patient-centred research project.

As we have argued so far and will be shown in the different chapters, our perspective is humanistic. However, we are aware of the emergence of machine translation and artificial intelligence in all areas of human communication. Although they are beyond the scope of this book, we have included in **Chapter 7** a few research issues that reflect current concerns regarding their use in patient-centred translation and communication.

There are unavoidable overlaps throughout the book. Due to their centrality, some concepts are recurrent (e.g. patient-centredness, patient's mother tongue, comprehensibility, empathy) and are approached in more than one chapter from different perspectives. Chapters 1 to 6 offer structured tasks that can be carried out both individually and in the classroom, as well as suggestions for tasks that can be further developed and adapted to the specific needs of different educational contexts. They also provide suggestions for further reading with a selected bibliography. Throughout the book, language-specific aspects have been avoided in the hope that most ideas can be extrapolated and adapted to the specific language or language combination of the translator, writer or health professional reading the book. To avoid heavy phrasing, when we use the word *communicators* we mean to include translators, interpreters, medical writers and health professionals.

Given the diverse audience with different disciplinary backgrounds that this book is aimed at, we recognise the value of including a basic glossary of language terms. This addition is intended to assist readers, particularly those from medicine and other health disciplines, by providing clarity and accessibility throughout the reading experience.

1

UNDERSTANDING CONTEXTS IN PATIENT-CENTRED COMMUNICATION

Overview of chapter

In this chapter, we provide a conceptual framework of relevant notions of context, some of which will be revisited and extended in practice in subsequent chapters. In contrast to biomedical research contexts, which are highly specialised and internationalised, patient-centred communication takes place in contexts and situations where specific cultures and languages play a crucial role. When translating and writing for patients, contexts can make translators and writers aware of the circumstances and values of individuals or groups of patients and can help them to respond appropriately to their needs and preferences.

The first contextual aspect we would like to highlight is patient-centred care and communication (Section 1.1), as this is the perspective we take in this book. In recent decades, the asymmetries of knowledge and power between patients and health professionals have given rise to new approaches that counterbalance the doctor-centred relationships that prevail in most health care settings. Person-centred approaches such as those of Carl Rogers have paved the way for the kind of humanised care, communication and translation that patient-centredness promotes. Context is essential because it provides the necessary framework for understanding the circumstances and meaning of messages exchanged between individuals. Words can have multiple interpretations, but context clarifies the specific meaning intended by the sender (Section 1.2). Finding and using contextual clues – distinguishing between the context of culture, in particular values about health and illness, and the context of situation, focusing on asymmetries between professionals and patients – and exploring the three dimensions of context can be useful in practical ways when translating and writing for patients.

DOI: 10.4324/9780429299698-2

With patients from different cultural backgrounds, awareness of cultural norms, customs and values can guide communicators to avoid cross-cultural misunderstandings and promote respectful interactions (Section 1.3). We understand culture in two complementary ways that are relevant to our patient-centred approach: culture in ethnic and national terms and culture in socio-professional terms. The fact that culture strongly influences communication as well as perceptions and conceptualisations of health should be acknowledged in the process of translating or writing for patients from different cultural backgrounds.

1.1 Understanding patient-centred communication

The word *patient* comes from Latin patī (suffer, bear, endure) + -nte(m), forming *patiente(m)*, which is a calque from Greek (Dicciomed). The Latin verb *patior* (to experience, undergo, endure) did not originally mean to be ill. The connotation of illness is a new meaning transferred from Greek páskhō πάσχω into Latin (Dicciomed), 'path' – (to suffer, and therefore to be ill), as in words such as pathogen, immunopathology or pathodontia in modern English and many other languages. Thus, etymologically, the word patient reflects a kind of passivity: someone to whom certain things happen, someone affected by certain negative health circumstances. Historically, patients have played passive, subordinate roles in their relationships with doctors and other health professionals, resulting in social and communicative asymmetries.

Doctor-centred approaches have traditionally dominated our understanding of medicine, health and clinical practice. The biomedical model on which doctors are trained at medical schools and act in clinical practice has been around since the mid-19th century. It focuses on the physical aspects of disease (such as anatomy, biochemistry, physiology, pathology and genetics) and adopts a positivist stance in its search for objective biomedical truth, mostly ignoring non-clinical factors regarding the individual patient's experience of illness. It leaves no room within its framework for the social, psychological and cultural dimensions of illness. In this context, Engel (1977) proposed a holistic, integrative biopsychosocial medical model to provide a blueprint for research, a framework for teaching and a design for action in the real world of health care.

1.1.1 The person-centred approach

In the field of care and communication, the clinical psychologist Carl Rogers (1995) developed his person-centred approach in the late 1950s, based on the principles and values of acceptance, caring, empathy and sensitivity in human interactions. He adopted the term *client*, not in the economic sense but as a person who relies on another for help and support and who seeks the professional advice or service of another. Based on this, he developed what he called the *person-centred approach to therapy*. His humanistic psychology was based on the idea that individuals have enormous resources for self-understanding and for changing their self-concepts, basic attitudes and self-directed behaviour and that these resources can be tapped if a definable climate of supportive psychological attitudes can be created (Rogers 1995). In subsequent decades, his ideas were used to frame other relationships between clients and the professionals they refer clients to, including learner-centred teaching and patient-centred care.

There are three conditions that must be present to facilitate a growth-promoting climate (Figure 1.1). The first one is genuineness, realness or congruence: when the therapist is transparent with the client, the relationship improves. The second is acceptance, caring or unconditional positive regard (Espstein et al. 2005). This means that the therapist has a positive and accepting attitude towards whatever the client is feeling. The third condition is empathic understanding, which involves sensitive, active listening. According to Rogers, fully accepting the patient as they are can be difficult, but it is also helpful. Trying to understand the person behind each of us – not just the words we say, but their meanings – genuinely and unconditionally caring for the individual and listening empathically are necessary conditions for effective and affective communication.

1) Genuineness, realness, transparency.
2) Acceptance, caring, prizing.
3) Empathic understanding, active listening, clarifying meaning.

FIGURE 1.1 The conditions of Roger's person-centred approach.

In recent decades, Roger's person-centredness evolved into patient-centredness, which describes a moral philosophy with three core values: 1) considering patients' needs, wants, perspectives and individual experiences; 2) providing opportunities for patients to contribute to and participate in their care; 3) enhancing partnership and understanding in the patient–doctor relationship (Espstein et al. 2005).

1.1.2 Patient-centredness

The term *patient-centred care* refers to patient-centred actions that focus on the following complementary areas (Little 2001): communication, partnership and health promotion. Patient-centred communication can be defined as a set of health professional skills demonstrated through verbal, paraverbal and non-verbal communication that facilitate patient-centred care (Hafskjold et al. 2015).

Empathy is considered a fundamental skill in all helping relationships, and the immediate outcomes of empathic communication are trust, mutual understanding, medication adherence, social support and self-efficacy (see Chapter 6). Mindfulness (the practice of deliberately focusing your attention on the present moment without judgment) and emotional intelligence (the ability to identify, express and regulate feelings and emotions in oneself and in others and to use feelings and emotions to motivate, plan and develop actions in clinical practice) are also relevant from a patient-centred perspective (Hafskjold et al. 2015). These communication skills enable health professionals to carry out the four basic actions we show in Figure 1.2 (Espstein et al. 2005).

1) Eliciting and understanding the patient's perspective – concerns, ideas, expectations, needs, feelings and functioning.
2) Understanding the patient in her or his unique psychosocial context.
3) Reaching a shared understanding of the problem and its treatment with the patient that is consistent with the patient's values.
4) Helping patients to share power and responsibility by involving them in decisions to the extent they wish.

FIGURE 1.2 Patient-centered communication: core actions.

Patient-centred care requires a therapeutic alliance; it involves agreement on goals and on interventions and an effective bond between patient and therapist. An individual's specific health needs and desired health outcomes are the driving force behind all health care decisions. Health care professionals treat patients not only clinically but also from emotional, mental, spiritual, social and cultural perspectives. Collaboration and shared decision-making between patients and health professionals are critical aspects of patient-centred care; emotional well-being is a top priority, along with physical comfort. Researchers found that vulnerable patients whether socioeconomically or because they are particularly unwell or distressed, show a strong preference for patient-centred care (Little 2001).

Communicators who deal with patients also need to acquire and develop empathy, mindfulness and emotional intelligence, and an accurate sense of patients' feelings and personal meanings can be very useful in patient communications. This is particularly important in face-to-face interactions, where both the health care professional and the interpreter can not only understand but also help to clarify patients' meanings. These can relate to personal feelings but also to cultural values reflected in language. For writers and translators, empathic understanding and clarifying meaning are equally important. As we show in Chapter 6, empathy and active listening can and should be incorporated into the tasks of both oral and written communication.

There are many factors that influence patient-centred communication (Epstein et al. 2005). Some are within the patient, such as previous illness, severity of current illness, emotional distress, personality, culture, values, family or socioeconomic status. Others are related to the health care system: access to care, choice of doctor, waiting times or institutional communication habits and preferences. Other factors are related to the doctor: personality, risk aversion, training or patient-centred versus doctor-centred orientation. Finally, the patient–doctor relationship itself is also a source of factors, including the duration of the relationship, the concordance of beliefs and values and issues of trust between patient and doctor (Espstein et al. 2005). In addition to these, we argue in this book that language plays a crucial role, particularly the patient's mother tongue (Montalt & García-Izquierdo 2002; Hemberg & Sved 2021; García-Izquierdo & Montalt 2022).

In recent decades, the patient-centred approach has been – and continues to be – developed in many health care systems because it can have important benefits for patients: better communication can improve satisfaction and clinical outcomes, and involving patients in partnership can have benefits without increasing their anxiety and with the potential to reduce adverse outcomes associated with prescribing (Little 2001). Although patient-centred care is not restricted to any particular medical specialty, it has gained particular prominence in reproductive health, home care, palliative care, gerontology and mental health. Patient-centred care can be applied in face-to-face consultations, where empathy, two-way communication and eye-to-eye contact are crucial. Patient-centred care can also be seen in hospitals where patients are given the choice to decide who can visit them and when and where family involvement is encouraged.

TASK 1.1 REFLECTING ON PATIENT-CENTREDNESS

Procedure

1) Read the following extracts from two medical websites aimed at patients and the public. They deal with the same condition: diabetic ketoacidosis.
2) Which do you think is more patient-centred? Why? Think about the strategies that make a text more or less patient-centred.

Materials

1) National Health Agency. UK National Health Service (NHS) website. Patient Services section, aimed at patients and the general public (Health A to Z section). www.nhs.uk/conditions/diabetic-ketoacidosis/
2) Hospital. Health Library section of Cedars-Sinai Hospital. www.cedars-sinai.org/health-library/diseases-and-conditions/d/diabetic-ketoacidosis.html

Text 1

Diabetic ketoacidosis

Diabetic ketoacidosis (DKA) is a serious problem that can occur in people with diabetes if their body starts to run out of insulin.

This causes harmful substances called ketones to build up in the body, which can be life-threatening if not spotted and treated quickly.

DKA mainly affects people with type 1 diabetes but can sometimes occur in people with type 2 diabetes. If you have diabetes, it's important to be aware of the risk and know what to do if DKA occurs.

Source: National Health Agency. UK National Health Service (NHS) website. Patient Services section, aimed at patients and the general public (Health A to Z section). www.nhs.uk/conditions/diabetic-ketoacidosis/

Treatments for diabetic ketoacidosis

DKA is usually treated in hospital. Treatments include:

- insulin, usually given into a vein
- fluids given into a vein to rehydrate your body
- nutrients given into a vein to replace any you've lost

You'll also be closely monitored for any life-threatening problems that can occur, such as problems with the brain, kidneys or lungs.

You can leave hospital when you're well enough to eat and drink and tests show a safe level of ketones in your body. It's normal to stay in hospital for a couple of days.

Before leaving hospital, ask to speak to a diabetes nurse about why DKA occurred and what you can do to stop it happening again.

Text 2

What is diabetic ketoacidosis?

Diabetic ketoacidosis (DKA) is a serious health problem that can happen if you have diabetes. It happens when chemicals called ketones build up in the blood.

Normally, the cells of your body take in and use sugar (glucose) as a source of energy. Glucose moves through the body in the blood. Insulin is a hormone that helps your cells take in the glucose from the blood. If you have diabetes, your cells can't take in and use this glucose in a normal way. This may be because your body doesn't make enough insulin. Or it may be because your cells don't respond to it normally.

As a result, glucose builds up in your blood and doesn't reach your cells. Without glucose to use, your body's cells burn fat instead of glucose for energy.

When cells burn fat, they make ketones. High levels of ketones can poison the body. High levels of glucose can also build up in your blood and cause other symptoms. Ketoacidosis also changes the amount of other substances in your blood. These include electrolytes such as sodium, potassium, and bicarbonate. This can lead to other problems.

Ketoacidosis happens most often in a person with type 1 diabetes. This is a condition where the body does not make enough insulin. In rare cases, ketoacidosis can happen in a person with type 2 diabetes. It can happen when they are under stress, such as when they are sick. Or when they have taken certain medicines that change how their bodies handle glucose.

DKA is pretty common. It is more common in younger people. Women have it more often than men.

How is diabetic ketoacidosis treated?

DKA needs to be treated right away in the hospital. Your healthcare provider will need to replace the large amount of fluids that you have lost. This is most often done through an IV.

You will also be given insulin. This will let your cells start using more glucose. This will help lower the levels of both ketones and sugar in your blood. You will likely also be given electrolytes, as these are often low as well.

If you have an illness that caused your ketoacidosis, your healthcare provider will treat that as well. For example, you may be given antibiotics for an infection.

You will need to have more blood tests during your treatment. This is so your healthcare provider can watch your condition and change your treatment as needed.

Source: Hospital. Health Library section of Cedars-Sinai Hospital. www.cedars-sinai.org/health-library/diseases-and-conditions/d/diabetic-ketoacidosis.html

Today, patient-centredness can also be seen at work even in biomedical fields such as personalised medicine, in which medications are often tailored to a patient's individual genetics, immune system, metabolism or biomarkers. Personalised medicines and therapies often require patient-centred communication strategies to ensure that partnership and health promotion at the individual level are achieved.

Patient-centredness is also relevant in pharmaceutical writing and translation, particularly in clinical trials for drug development involving patients. In these contexts, summaries for patients are produced to adequately inform participants about the results of given clinical trials (see Chapter 2 for a detailed description of this genre). Many of these are originally written in English and then translated into other languages.

Alternatively, local versions of summaries for patients may be written and produced originally in the language of the patients. Using the patients' language and being culturally sensitive are some of the key challenges in patient-centred communication in clinical trials. For example, Mogami et al. (2017) determined that locally developed summaries for patients in Japanese were more patient-centred than those translated from other languages, bringing more benefits to both patients and the pharmaceutical industry. This seems to be also the case in more culturally and linguistically diverse regions such as the European Union. Another important concept in the pharmaceutical context is patient centricity, which entails designing treatments, clinical trials or other health solutions with the patient in mind. This is not a new concept, but it is becoming increasingly important in regulatory documents (James & Bharadia 2019).

Suggestions for task. Patient-centredness versus patient-centricity

Explore the similarities and differences between patient-centredness and patient-centricity. Kialo (www.kialo.com/), a web-based tool for exploring controversial topics, can help you address and problematise the issue of whether patients should have a more proactive role as in patient-centred care and communication or a more passive one as in patient-centric care and communication.

You can read this article where patient centricity is defined: Yeoman, G.; Furlong, P.; Seres, M.; Binder, H.; Chung, H.; Garzya, V.; Jones, R.R. Defining patient centricity with patients for patients and caregivers: A collaborative endeavour. *BMJ Innov.* **2017**, 3, 76–83. https://innovations.bmj.com/content/3/2/76

The patient-centred approach is widely advocated as a quality model in many health systems, but its implementation in practice is still limited and uneven for several reasons. The first being time constraints. Health professionals often complain that they don't have enough time to establish patient-centred interactions in face-to-face or distance consultations. Second, the lack of formal, academic training of health professionals in communication and cultural competence has a negative impact on the way they communicate with patients. In addition, lifelong learning is poor or non-existent in many health systems, which does not help health professionals who wish to improve their communication skills. Third, some health professionals lack not only the appropriate training but also the appropriate attitudes towards patient-centredness. Fourth, it is not easy to combine evidence-based, disease-oriented approaches with patient-centred approaches that focus on the individual experience of illness. Finally, language and cultural barriers play a negative role in patient-centred care.

1.1.3 Patient-centred translation

In care settings, language is much more than a tool for communication because of its important emotional dimension (Hemberg & Sved 2021). Patients find it easier both to provide relevant information to health professionals and to express their feelings and emotions in their mother tongue. It is also easier for them to understand relevant written and oral information provided by health professionals in their own language.

Translating in a patient-centred way means, firstly, addressing the patient in their own language, either directly or through a translator; it also means encouraging them to express themselves in that language. Information and knowledge asymmetries between health professionals and patients increase dramatically when they do not share the same language and culture. If linguistic and cultural barriers are not addressed appropriately and professionally, they can lead to impaired caring relationships, inequality, vulnerability and exclusion. Research has shown that the more serious the illness, the more important it is for patients to be able to express themselves in their mother tongue (Hemberg & Sved 2021) (see Chapter 4).

We argue that language is at the heart of patient care, and in today's multi-ethnic societies where multilingual and multicultural communities and interactions abound, translation really matters. Patient-centred translation (Montalt 2017) refers to a type of user-centred translation (Suojanen et al. 2015) that focuses on the perspective of the target patient (Figure 1.3). It aims to achieve full patient comprehension (see Chapter 5), empathy (see Chapter 6), empowerment and well-being through grammatical, terminological, stylistic, textual and pragmatic means in the patient's mother tongue, as well as through non-verbal resources. It takes into account the

- Patient's mother tongue.
- Relevance and meaningfulness.
- Comprehensibility.
- Empathy – person-first language, etc.
- Awareness of context and situation.
- Awareness of cultural differences and health pluralism.
- Professionalism in translation tasks.
- Ethics – respect, inclusiveness, equality, etc.
- Trust in interlingual and intercultural translation/mediation.
- Accessibility and multimodality.

FIGURE 1.3 Main domains of patient-centred translation (Montalt 2017) (including interpreting and writing).

educational background, clinical situation, specific needs and preferences of both individual and well-defined subgroups of patients in the presentation of information.

In patient-centred translation, the individual patient's context and specific situation are paramount; it is an emotionally supportive, culturally relevant and coherent process. Therefore, the patient's mother tongue is central, and intralingual translation is a fundamental component, as efforts must be made to ensure that the register is adequate in addition to the patient's mother tongue. Patient-centred translation relies and depends on constant testing and feedback from real target patients (Montalt 2017).

How we treat patients starts with how we talk or write about or to them. Choices about language use shape how individuals think, feel and behave towards others, including people with disabilities (Crocker & Smith 2019). Emphasising their individuality and personhood, rather than their impairments or conditions empowers patients. For example, *chronic pain patients* emphasises the condition of chronic pain as a characteristic of patients, whereas *patients with chronic pain* more clearly separates the person from the condition. Other examples are much more disrespectful: compare *retarded* versus *having intellectual disabilities*. Writing and translating for patients in a patient-centred way means being aware of these linguistic issues and their emotional consequences and avoiding stigmatisation and derogatory descriptions (see Chapter 6).

1.2 Exploring context

Context is crucial in patient-centred communication. In this section, we explain how context affects communication with patients, define types of context and present the categories that determine the so-called dimensions of context, which are essential when writing, translating and interpreting for patients.

Systemic functional linguistics (Eggins 2004) is a social theory of language that is strongly influenced by the theory of situational context proposed by the anthropologist Malinowski, who was one of the first scholars to carry out fieldwork. He was associated with functionalism in anthropology, which held that each of the components and social institutions of a system fulfils a function. As early as 1923, Malinowski argued that in order to understand a text (or a communicative utterance), it was necessary to place it in its verbal and non-verbal environment and to consider more than the words themselves.

Systemic functional linguistics theories were also inspired by Firth's theory of context-dependent function (Firth 1935), which stressed the importance of knowing how to interpret the intended meaning of an utterance as well as the literal meaning of the words. An example in the medical field is hospitals, where medical staff often use informal language in the form of jargon (Navarro 2012) – such as abbreviations, humour, puns, metonymy and metaphors – because it has great expressive power to refer to different procedures, to talk about subjects that are taboo (such as cancer or death) or to help understand each other more quickly. Translators and interpreters often struggle to understand and mediate in these situations, and contextual cues can be of great help.

In the 1970s, proponents of Systemic functional linguistics (Hasan 1985) used these theories as a starting point to define context in cultural terms as "an integrated body of the total set of meanings available to a community: its semiotic potential" (Halliday & Hasan 1985/1989: 99), as we will see in the last section of this chapter. For its part, the field of sociolinguistics recognises that one of the aims of linguistic analysis is to describe communicative events in context. Some authors (Cook-Gumperz & Gumperz 1976; Gumperz 1992) propose that participants in a communicative event must be able to guide each other's interpretations of what is said. In these studies, the scholars refer to the mental processes that enable participants in a communicative event to evoke the cultural background and social expectations necessary to interpret speech.

Gumperz (1992) relates the concepts of *understanding* and *contextualisation*: speakers' and listeners' use of verbal and non-verbal signs to link what is said at any one time and in any one place with knowledge acquired through past experience. He argues for the existence of contextualisation cues such as stress and intonation as well as paralinguistic features including tempo and laughter, choice of code and particular lexical expressions. These cues are language specific, and their inappropriate use in inter- or cross-cultural communication can lead to serious misunderstandings whose origins are difficult to trace (Couper-Kuhlen 2019).

Gumperz's theory, which was originally conceived to explain oral interactions, can also be applied to written texts, as there will also be genre conventions (see Chapter 2) that allow recipients to evoke previous experiences. For example, we can interpret a patient information leaflet based on contextualisation cues. In this case, these cues are not related to intonation and paralinguistics but to textual cohesion mechanisms such as deixis or pronominal references, lexis and terminology and connectors, to mention a few, which will help the reader to interpret the text correctly. As we can see in Figure 1.4, which corresponds to the first section of a patient information leaflet, we can find various cohesion mechanisms: directives or imperatives to show the relevance of actions (e.g. *read, keep, ask, do not pass on*), a personal approach to address the reader directly (*you start taking, if you have any further questions, your doctor*, etc.) and adverbs to emphasise important actions (*carefully*).

Package leaflet. Information for the user

Read all of this leaflet carefully before you start taking this medicine because it contains important information for you.

- Keep this leaflet. You may need to read it again.
- If you have any further questions, ask your doctor or pharmacist.
- Do not pass this medicine on to others. It may harm them, even if their signs of illness are the same as yours.

If you get any side effects, talk to your doctor or pharmacist. This includes any possible side effects not listed in this leaflet.

FIGURE 1.4 Excerpt of a patient information leaflet.

The concept of contextualisation will therefore be crucial for writing, translating or interpreting the content of oral or written communication. In the case of medical communication, we also encounter a rich, dynamic continuum from interactions between experts in highly specialised research journals to news in the press about health and medicine. This means that both the participants in the different communicative events and the contexts in which they take place can be very diverse. However, the pandemic situation we experienced in 2020 forced international health authorities to plan communication processes on a global scale, with public health campaigns aimed at the world's population. This meant that specific contexts were sometimes overlooked.

Each country's health care system is unique, but even within the same country, there are obvious differences between systems that can have different regulations on procedures and patient relations. Additionally, in most countries, a public health care system coexists with a private one that, although regulated by the same laws, usually has more resources and more flexible procedures for providing patient care.

In multilingual societies, there is also the problem of not providing translation and interpretating services in minority languages, which means that health care is not provided in some patient's mother tongues. In the European context, this is highlighted in the European Commission's report on studies on translation and multilingualism (Angelelli 2015), which emphasises that without consolidated legislation in the different countries, in the absence of formal language services and "in the absence of a common language, professional language provision is central not only to cross-border healthcare, but also to communication in healthcare in general (as well as in all other areas of public services) in each MS [Member State] of the EU" (Angelelli 2015). This report emphasises that in most cases "there is no consistent provision of translation documents needed for cross-border healthcare [...] and in practice the responsibility for translation of all documents is placed on the patient" (Angelelli 2015: 91).

Given that linguistic diversity is a defining characteristic of the European Union, this report recommends that legislation on language provision and quality be harmonised. It also recommends that language service providers be included as part of the health care team. This would mean that health professionals could benefit from language service providers in working with culturally diverse patients. Discussion of linguistic/cultural diversity and communication should be included in the curricula for students at medical schools. Alternatively, the report suggests possibly assembling a register of professional and certified translators and interpreters working in health care settings.

1.2.1 Context of culture and context of situation

The initial, more orthodox view of Systemic functional linguistics was revised and extended by the representatives of the so-called Sidney School (Martin 1992) and applied by scholars of textual approaches in linguistics and translation studies (Hatim & Mason 1990, 1997; Swales 1990; Biber 1995; Biber & Conrad 2019), who believe that the context plays a decisive role in the choice of grammatical and lexical units by the author or translator at the decision-making stage. For the Sidney School, it is also necessary to stratify the context into coexisting layers:

- The context of culture, that is "the environment in which meanings are exchanged", in which the different textual manifestations of the genre are interpreted (Halliday & Webster 2009).
- The context of situation refers to the specific context in which a text is framed and in which the text genre (see Chapter 2) is realised. It is the second level of realisation in which the register and its categories are manifested: the field or sphere of interaction (which includes the subject matter); the mode or modality of exchange, and the tenor or level of formality, from the colloquial to the academic.

Taking the patient information leaflet as a case in focus, the field is medical (and the subject matter varies according to the medicine and disease in question); the medium can be a printed document, a website or an app for instance; and the tenor is formal but directly addressed to the reader. It is often socially and geographically unmarked and can – or should – be understandable by an averagely literate population.

Another example is the living will, a standardised and routine genre in many cultures but one which can be actualised in different ways: in this case, the field is medical-legal and the subject is a person's wishes regarding medical treatment at the end of life. However, there may be significant differences in its mode (orally, in the presence of a notary or by means of a recording; handwritten; drawn up on a computer, etc.) and, above all, in its tenor, if no standardised model is used, since the degree of formality will depend on the patient's level of education, age or other personal factors.

The context in which medical communication is produced may be highly institutionalised, such as a hospital or a health centre, or outside the health system altogether, as in the case of an individual patient finding information about a disease from a book or website. In all cases, the context regulates the nature of the communication and allow us to identify whether or not the communicative exchange is taking place in an appropriate way.

From a translation-oriented functionalist perspective, Hatim and Mason (1990) argue that context is organised in three broad dimensions:

- Textual: the grammatical and lexical mechanisms that make a text consistent.
- Communicative: who is being addressed and in what specific situation; the register; the pragmatic mechanisms used – speech acts such as affirming, denying, questioning, doubting – and the information assumed to be shared between sender and receiver.
- Cognitive: the conceptual content of the text, the ideology conveyed, the degree of readability or comprehensibility (see Chapter 5) and the accessibility necessary in any communicative exchange.

Only by adequately interpreting all the contextual aspects involved in these three dimensions will the communicator be able to adequately convey the message of the original text and meet the expectations of the addressees.

1.3 The concept of culture in patient-centred communication

It is often assumed that sharing a language is enough to ensure understanding, but this is not often the case, as misunderstandings can also occur due to cultural differences. Culture is a paramount factor in understanding communication contexts and audiences (see Chapter 4). Given the increasing need to provide health services to patients from different cultures and languages, it is essential to recognise culture as a crucial element of health and illness. In this section, we will focus on how culture influences communication, what the culture-specific ways of communicating are, and what health-related issues can be influenced – negatively – by cultural differences.

1.3.1 Defining culture

In the literature, we can find many definitions and approaches to the concept of culture from different perspectives: anthropology, psychology, communication, applied linguistics, etc. (for detailed reviews, see e.g. Hua 2014; Katan 2018; Grainger & Mills 2016 or Katan & Taibi 2021). Most scholars seem to agree that culture comprises a shared set of attitudes, values, goals, beliefs, rituals, practices and forms of expression that characterise a particular group of people and evolve over time.

In this context, a group of people should be understood in a broad sense. Although the understanding is still predominantly as referring only to race/ethnicity and national belonging, by group we also refer to the following:

- Religious groups (Buddhism, Christianity, Hinduism, Islam, Judaism, etc.) that may influence the worldview, ethics and lifestyle of their members.
- Organisations that have their own culture, structure, leadership style, goals, size and history.
- Professional groups; each profession has its own culture.
- Communities of practice, whose members, united by a common enterprise, share a common domain of interest and engage in common activities and practices (Hua 2014: 188–189).

As we can see, culture is a very broad concept and refers to the beliefs, values and practices of *any* social group that may be considered a community. In addition to these considerations about culture, we highlight defining culture in socio-professional terms (Montalt & Shuttleworth 2012). Socio-professional cultures are relevant to this book because patients are the community of practice, as opposed to that of health professionals (Montalt & García-Izquierdo 2024). Culture can range from people belonging to certain ethnic groups (Italians, Latin Americans, Chinese, etc.) to a group that comes together because they share certain characteristics or situations (e.g. patients suffering from the same disease and receiving the same treatment). These cultural groups articulate communication through text genres, which may vary from one culture to another. Genres are also influenced by other factors that may intersect with the group, such as the gender or age of the members. In Chapter 2, we will return to the concept of genre and illustrate all these aspects.

In today's globalised world, cultures are in constant evolution, and people, especially those involved in migration processes, may have to adapt culturally at different points in their lives. Despite these changes and overlaps, there are some aspects rooted in the culture of origin that continue to strongly influence different facets of daily life, with illness and treatment being among the most influential (CRIT 2009; Neubauer et al. 2015). As Crezee (2013) point out, even people who migrated to another country many years ago and feel that they have assimilated into their new country in many aspects of their lives may revert to their original cultural attitudes when faced with illness.

Therefore, when translating, writing and interpreting, it is essential to have cultural awareness of health, which includes an understanding of how a person's culture may influence their values, behaviours, beliefs and basic assumptions about health-related issues (Neubauer et al. 2015). It should be noted, however, that attributing differences and variations in communication styles to cultural values carries the risk of stereotyping, which should be avoided. For example, stating that patients of Chinese origin may behave in a certain way should not be equated with stating that an individual patient in a medical consultation will inevitably behave in such a way because they were born in China (CRIT 2009).

1.3.2 Influence of culture on communication

Culture influences communication in different ways, and what is appropriate in one culture may be perceived in a very different way in another. The literature on intercultural mediation and interpreting in public services has provided us with a wide range of studies on how culture influences the way we interact (CRIT 2009; Ji et al. 2019), in particular:

- The amount of information embedded in the context, which influences the degree of explicitness or implicitness of the information provided.
- The content of the message and the way it is delivered (i.e. the degree of directness and the use of non-verbal aspects).
- The paralinguistic aspects (tone of voice, speed of delivery, intonation, length of pauses, to name but a few).

High- vs low-context cultures and degree of explicitness

Cultures can be classified according to the amount of explicit verbal information that members of a culture use in their communicative interactions. According to Hall (1976), there are differences in the extent to which the meaning of a message comes primarily from the context or from the utterances themselves. The more a culture relies on context in communication, the less it communicates information explicitly; such cultures are called high context and some examples are China, Japan, Thailand or Brazil; in communications in these cultures, contextual cues relevant to interpreting messages include social status, social relationships, environment or non-verbal behaviour. Conversely, low-context cultures are less dependent on context, preferring directness and explicit information, such as Germany, Sweden and the United States. Communicators need to be aware of the degree of explicitness or implicitness of oral and written genres in particular cultures: some patients will need information to be very explicit and detailed, while others will be able to use the context of the communication to infer meaning and therefore need less detailed information (Byrne 2014).

Degree of directness and power distance

The degree of directness/indirectness is linked to the concept of high/low-context cultures. Hall (1998: 61) argues that

> high context communication or message is one in which most of the information is already in the person, while very little is in the coded, explicit, transmitted part of the message. A low-context communication is just the opposite, that is, the mass of the information is vested in the explicit code.

Directness can also be influenced by the topic of communication: with sensitive topics such as life-threating illnesses or aggressive treatments, even low-context cultures sometimes use more indirect language. This means that neither directness/indirectness nor high/low-context cultures are absolute concepts. Rather, we need to think of a continuum linking the two extremes along which the different cultural groups can be placed. Cultural attitudes towards authority and power distance can influence the degree of directness and formality with which information is presented. The concept of power distance explains how members of a group respond to what they perceive to be an authority figure, and doctors are seen as authorities in many cultures and are addressed in very indirect, formal and subordinate ways.

Taboo topics

Many cultures have topics that are considered taboo and tend to be avoided, usually relating to sex, death or mental health. For example, Ortí et al. (2006) and CRIT (2009) studied, respectively, populations in the Maghreb and in western Africa and found that both usually avoid talking about sex in public settings and in asymmetric communicative situations such as medical consultations. Interpreters should be aware of the potential pitfalls of this aspect of patient–doctor interactions and even intervene to warn that something may be a taboo subject in the patient's culture (Crezee & Roat 2019). By the same token, patients might misunderstand or even reject a written information leaflet about sex provided in a clinical setting if the issue is not addressed sensitively.

Non-verbal communication

Non-verbal language includes eye contact, physical proximity, body contact, facial expressions and hand gestures. Cultural differences are particularly evident in non-verbal language and communicative interaction patterns, which can differ between health professionals and patients even when they speak the same language.

There are many examples of how non-verbal language can lead to misunderstandings if not dealt with appropriately. For example, in cultures such as India and Pakistan, it is considered disrespectful and aggressive to look doctors in the eye, and it is preferable to look at them from the corner of the eye (CRIT 2009). In other cultures, this may be interpreted as not listening to the doctor. Regarding physical contact, in some cultures people refuse to be touched by health professionals during physical examinations, while in others, patients expect to be touched, believing that physical contact is essential for a correct diagnosis. In terms of physical proximity, there are cultures in which members move very close to the health professional they are talking to and may find it very offensive if they move back to gain more physical space. Emotional recognition can also vary across cultures. Although it is generally assumed that facial expressions of emotion communicate the same feelings everywhere, each culture may have different expectations about when, how, where and to whom facial expressions are displayed (Hua 2014).

Paralinguistic aspects

Paralinguistic features (such as loudness, tone, speed, pausing or turn taking) also play an indispensable role in the way a spoken message is interpreted, especially when the listener and the speaker do not share the same cultural background. For example, speaking in a very low voice expresses respect in some cultures, whereas in others it may be interpreted as a sign of shyness. The length of pauses between turns can also be problematic: in some cultures, doctors are expected to take turns and patients to take long pauses as a sign of respect. However, these long pauses may be interpreted by members of other cultures as a sign of hesitation or lack of understanding. Before interpreting, interpreters should ask themselves whether there are any gestures, postures, facial expressions or paralinguistic aspects of the patients that might be misunderstood by health professionals from other backgrounds and vice versa. It is worth pointing out that interpreters have a clarifying role and can intervene in their own voice or in a follow-up session (Angelelli 2008).

1.3.3 Culture and health

Just as they differ in many other areas, different cultures have different beliefs, values and attitudes about health and illness that can strongly influence the interpretation of symptoms, the understanding of illness and the expectations about treatment and compliance (Napier et al. 2014). Some of the most culturally sensitive areas are sexual health, pregnancy and labour, death, end of life situations or the expression of pain.

Gynaecology and obstetrics is one of the medical specialties most sensitive to cultural differences. For example, there are cultures in which women have long periods of rest during pregnancy, which conflicts with what health professionals in other cultures consider most appropriate for a healthy pregnancy. In some Asian cultures, following the philosophy of yin and yang, women usually follow a special diet during pregnancy and after childbirth, even though this may interfere with medically prescribed treatments. Infertility can also be a source of difference, as there are cultures where it is widely frowned upon and seen as a woman's problem – and even a reason for rejection by the husband or partner. This can cause significant problems if the issue arises during a medical consultation.

In some cultures, patients are not told directly that they have a terminal illness and instead the bad news is given to whoever is considered the head of the family – usually the father or eldest son. Other cultures generally oppose autopsies and organ donation after death because of the importance of preserving the integrity of the body. Attitudes towards pain can also vary greatly in different cultures. Patients in some cultures express their pain by screaming, shouting and moaning, believing that by doing so they are asking relatives and friends to visit them. Some other cultures, either because they follow a principle of conflict avoidance or because they value self-control and self-restraint, tend not to express their pain in public. If not interpreted correctly, both situations can lead to misdiagnosis by health care professionals.

The translator/interpreter needs to anticipate situations where different cultural attitudes to health and illness may lead to misunderstandings and non-compliance with health professionals' instructions if they are contrary to certain cultural beliefs. For this reason, it is important to be familiar with the cultural background of both the patient and the health professional, as well as the beliefs and practices underlying the health care system in which the patient–doctor interaction takes place. The notion of medical pluralism can be useful in responding to different worldviews about health and illness (Perdiguero 2004). According to Khalikova (2020, 2023), medical pluralism describes the availability of different approaches, treatments and institutions that people in different cultures use to maintain health or treat illness. Most commonly, medical pluralism involves the use of Western medicine (or *biomedicine*) and what is variously called *traditional medicine* and *alternative medicine*, such as traditional Chinese medicine, Ayurvedic medicine or homeopathy.

Suggestions for task. Reflect on your own culture

Have you ever experienced or directly witnessed any communication problems due to cultural differences in health? How were or could these problems have been resolved?

As we have seen in this section, the way we communicate about health and illness is deeply influenced by culture. In the next chapter, we will look at some of the most common genres used in medical and health settings, and we will see that some are more standardised internationally than others. However, all text genres are the result of complex social and cultural processes and are socially and culturally embedded. They are recognised as genres and make sense to readers/users only in specific contexts.

Further reading

Angelelli, C. V. *Medical Interpreting and Cross-Cultural Communication*; Cambridge University Press: Cambridge, 2024.

Crezee, I. *Introduction to Healthcare for Interpreters and Translators*; John Benjamins Publishing Company: Amsterdam; Philadelphia, 2013.

Hua, Z. *Exploring Intercultural Communication: Language in Action*; Routledge. Routledge Introductions to Applied Linguistics: Oxon; New York, 2014.

Jiang, S.; Wu, Z.; Zhang, X.; Ji, Y.; Xu, J.; Liu, P.; Chen, J. How Does Patient-Centered Communication Influence Patient Trust? The Roles of Patient Participation and Patient Preference. *Patient Education and Counseling*, 2024, 108161.

Montalt, V. Patient-Centred Translation and Emerging Trends in Medicine and Health Care. *European Society for Translation Studies (EST) Newsletter*, 2017, *51*, 10–11.

Parthab Taylor, S.; Nicolle, C.; Maguire, M. Cross-Cultural Communication Barriers in Health Care. *Nursing Standard*, 2013, *27* (31), 135.

Pinto, R. Z.; Ferreira, M. L.; Oliveira, V. C.; Franco, M. R.; Adams, R.; Maher, C. G.; Ferreira, P. H. Patient-Centred Communication is Associated with Positive Therapeutic Alliance: A Systematic Review. *Journal of Physiotherapy*, 2012, *58* (2), 77–87.
Rogers, C. R. *A Way of Being*; Houghton Mifflin Harcourt, 1995.
Suojanen, T.; Koskinen, K.; Tuominen, T. *User-Centered Translation*; Routledge: London, 2014.

2

DIVERSITY OF TEXT GENRES FOR PATIENTS

Overview of chapter

Communication in health care settings is articulated through genres. This chapter uses the notion of text genre as a conceptual framework to explore the characteristics and conventions of some of the most common genres in which patients are involved, both as target readers/users and as actual writers/addressers (Section 2.1). Getting to know these genres well – their communicative purposes, the situations in which they are used, the motivations and expectations of their participants and their typical structure and form – is key to successful communication, both intra- and interlingually.

Paying attention to the conventions of the genre is a key aspect when writing the target text. Even if it belongs to the same genre as the source text, there may be important differences in the way it is realised in the target language and culture. Genres can also be used to bridge the gap between users of the same language who belong to different discourse communities (i.e. doctors and patients). These genres can be described as reformulations and re-contextualisations of more specialised genres, such as original articles or medical treatises.

In this chapter, we introduce Olivia (Section 2.2), a fictional character who uses some of the genres presented and who will accompany us throughout the rest of the book to illustrate some of the key aspects of patient-centred translation and communication. Genres covered in detail in this chapter include patient information leaflets, fact sheets for patients, summaries for patients, informed consent forms, medical reports, patient narratives and patient-reported outcomes. Special attention is also given to emerging genres such as mobile apps and comics (Section 2.3).

DOI: 10.4324/9780429299698-3

2.1 The concept of genre

At some point in our lives, most of us will need to seek medical help in a primary care centre. This involves putting in a request (by telephone, in-person, or online) and receiving confirmation. At the health centre on the day of the appointment, we are asked for documentation so that the doctor can see us and, depending on our complaint, prescribe medication or ask us to undergo diagnostic tests (a blood test, a CAT scan, an MRI scan, etc.). Carrying out these tests will entail the need for authorisations as well as subsequent reports being sent to the consultant. In most cultural and linguistic communities, these texts serve a variety of communicative purposes and are aimed at specific target groups whom we recognise as members of that community. These different kinds of texts are generally called *genres* and have been widely acknowledged in the last century or so. In any community, these different genres are routinely used and easily recognised as appropriate in specific contexts as part of a received heritage and associated with given communicative situations.

Genres manifest themselves in different degrees of formality and of speciality (registers). A recipe, an obituary, an opinion article, a comic, a short story, a poster, a complaint, an instruction manual, a forensic report, a research article, a summary for patients, a patient information leaflet or a clinical guideline are examples of genres. Genre is a rich, complex concept that helps writers and translators relate the text to its context of production and connects different relevant dimensions (García-Izquierdo 2011): text, communication, and cognition (see subsection 1.2.2 in Chapter 1). We need to consider these aspects as permeable compartments (Aragonés 2009; Borja et al. 2009) that need to be analysed jointly if we wish to understand them. This richness is precisely what makes genre a central notion in the field of intralingual and interlingual communication.

Genres are therefore relevant categories for any discursive community, whether it be professional or not. Genre is not to be confused with type of text, which refers to the predominant rhetorical function of texts, such as instruction, argumentation or description (Hatim & Mason 1990) Thus, we can talk about predominantly instructive (e.g. patient information leaflet), argumentative (e.g. opinion article) and descriptive (e.g. forensic report) genres. Genres can also be addressed to different recipients, and medical genres are no exception: within the medical field, we find some addressed to specialists and others addressed to or produced by patients (see types of patients in Chapter 4), which are the ones we will focus on in this chapter.

Most genres are highly conventionalised and are constructed in a prototypical way that is reflected in recurrent structures. However, the level of routinisation of a given genre can vary within the same culture. There are highly routinised genres (such as the patient information leaflet, which is even regulated by the European Medicines Agency) but also those that are more flexible in their structural and linguistic conventions, such as the patient narrative, as we shall see.

To these variations between genres within the same language must be added those that occur between languages and cultures (genres that do not exist in some cultures, or that exist but show different conventions regarding structure, style, register or terminological usage), which can cause mismatches. This is a challenge for translators, who need to use different strategies and justifies the relevance of genre competence (Montalt & García-Izquierdo 2002); that is, the ability to predict the genre organisation of a text in a given language and culture and make the necessary adjustments to adequately link it to the communicative situation and context. A genre approach to translating and communication enables us to generate more acceptable texts from the point of view of the community that receives them.

2.1.1 Grouping genres in different ways

We will now consider the difficulty of determining to what extent some genres are linked to and depend on each other (this is called *intertextuality*). Take reports as an example. There are different types of reports in different fields: special examination report, consultation report or preoperative report, just to mention a few. In this example, report is the genre and the different kinds of reports are subgenres (Bhatia 1993). There are also supra-genres that encompass multiple independent genres, such as medical records or histories: the full record of information about a person's health – diagnoses, medicines, tests, allergies, immunisations, and treatment plans – with emphasis on the events affecting the patient during a specific care episode. Complete medical records will contain multiple genres, such as the discharge report, the informed consent form or the pathology report.

Another way of exploring interdependence between genres is focusing on how separate genres are functionally linked with or derived from other genres. In this regard, the concept of genre system is especially useful for analysing and understanding complex communication in medical and health settings. *Genre systems* (Bazerman 1994) or *repertoires of genres* (Orlikowski & Yates 1994a, 1994b; Yates & Orlikowski 2002) are clusters of interdependent genres represented in typically related sequences. A genre system includes the sequences in which one genre follows another in a typical communication flow of a given group of people (Bazerman 2003). An example is the system made up of the genres in which a patient is involved, from the time the patient goes to the general practitioner and is recommended to be admitted to hospital for surgery, until they are discharged from the hospital. Another example of a genre system is the process from empirical research to clinical practice, which is channeled through several genres (see a visual representation of such a genre system in Montalt & González-Davies 2007: 65).

Another closely related concept is that of *genre ecology* (Spinuzzi et al. 2000), which refers to the interconnectedness of genres that have differentiating conventions working in unison to address a single topic to a broad audience. An example are the campaigns performed in different countries during the Covid-19 pandemic by public health authorities. These range from official and regulatory documents (e.g. vaccination strategies or minutes of meetings of technical committees) to infographics, videos, podcasts and other informative-didactic materials on keys to protect oneself from the virus, how to act in the event of symptoms or how to use a mask.

Finally, we can group genres according to their shared overall purpose. For example, university textbooks or clinical cases used in medical schools are examples of genres used in a pedagogical context. This way of grouping texts is what we call *genre colonies* (Bhatia 2014), that is, groups of closely related genres that clearly respond to similar – but not necessarily identical – communicative purposes such as educating and training future medical professionals. These genres often belong to the same disciplinary field.

We should consider that any attempt to establish a classification of genres will necessarily be limited (García-Izquierdo 2009) because genres are dynamic; they evolve historically and culturally. There are emerging ones (e.g. a medical app), as we shall see in this chapter, while some of the canonical ones (e.g. a handwritten report) are disappearing. Translators and communicators must develop, in parallel to the translating and communicative competence, their multilingual and multicultural generic competence, which will define their professional identity and will be crucial in practice to act as an interlingual and intercultural communicator (García-Izquierdo & Montalt 2013) and to face restrictions of various kinds that must be resolved with the appropriate strategies.

To perform their work properly, like in their educational and training stages, writers and translators should ask themselves a series of questions related to the aspects we have explained, which are summarised in Figure 2.1. by the GENTT Research Group (Textual Genres for Translation, www.gentt.uji.es) at the Universitat Jaume I, Spain.

Suggestions for task. Exploring genre

Using the minicorpus of patient-centred genres you can find on the Routledge Translation Studies Portal, explore the following questions:

- Which context and specific situation do you think each of the texts is used in?
- Who has written each of the texts?
- For which purpose?
- How is the purpose and intention of the text manifested in the language?
- Who reads each of the texts?
- Why?
- What for?
- Will the reader need to use the information for practical reasons?
- Which information?

Compare each of these texts in English with similar texts in your target language. How do they differ in terms of formal structure, register, style, communicative function and cognitive orientation?

GENRE (Name)	
OTHER NAMES	
DEFINITION	
COMMUNICATIVE SITUATION	Register: socio-professional field, mode, level of formality Participants: sender(s), receivers(s) Function
SUB-GENRE	If applicable
EQUIVALENT GENRE (in other languages)	
RELATION WITH OTHER GENRES (genres systems)	
FORMAL ASPECTS	Grammatical cohesion, such as collocations, deixis and ellipsis Lexical cohesion, such as terminological, phraseological and semantic aspects
LEGAL FRAMEWORK	Normative texts that may apply
MACROSTRUCTURE/MOVES	Identification of the main parts of the text
COMMENTS	Relevant sources of information about the genre

FIGURE 2.1 Genre analysis template proposed by the GENTT research group.

2.2 Introducing Olivia, our patient

Let us now imagine a patient for whom we write or translate. Her name is Olivia. She is our patient. Olivia has just been to visit the doctor. In the consultation, the doctor has prescribed a drug that will hopefully help her in a safe and effective way. She must take the medicine at the right time and in the right quantities. If she does not, the medicine will probably not work and, what is worse, could harm her. The doctor has told her how the medicine works and how to take it, but she will not remember, so she needs a written piece of text to remember the relevant information about the medicine she is supposed to take. This vital information is provided in the patient information leaflet.

To manage her condition, Olivia needs information beyond that provided in the patient information leaflet for a particular medicine, such as the cause of her disease, its symptoms, its risk factors, its complications, its available treatments or what changes in her lifestyle could help her. She may also want information about support groups she can join to share her experience and learn from others. All this general information about a particular disease can be found in fact sheets for patients.

Olivia is a very active patient and a person full of curiosity about what is going on with her health, and she may also want to know about how researchers are advancing their understanding of her condition as well as any new treatment available. That is why she would like to read relevant state-of-the-art research. The problem is that this type of information is available in highly specialised articles that researchers publish in biomedical journals. Some of them are starting to publish simplified versions addressed to patients who, like Olivia, would like to understand more about her disease and the prospects of finding a good course of treatment for it. These are called summary for patients.

Olivia will soon have to undergo surgery as part of her therapeutic plan that she and her doctor have explored and agreed on. Surgical operations often involve risks, and for Olivia to decide whether she wants to run them and understand the balance between risks and benefits, she needs to discuss the situation with someone who really knows the procedure in a detailed way. In many health care systems, Olivia's decision must be signed in a written document that has legal value. This is called the informed consent form.

During her therapeutic process, Olivia often receives medical information about herself and the progression of her disease. For example, when she has a blood test, an x-ray scan or a biopsy, she often has access to and can read what the specialist has written in the medical report. These reports are addressed to other doctors, not to patients, and tend to be written in specialised language. More and more, patients like Olivia wish to enhance their autonomy and want to understand these documents about themselves and be able to make sense of them.

Increasingly, companies in the medical and health sectors try to meet their clients' needs and increase their satisfaction rates. Recently, Olivia has been asked to participate in a survey with the aim to improve the lives of patients taking a particular drug. For this purpose, they use a patient self-report tool called a patient report of outcomes, a report of the status of patients' health condition or health behaviour that comes directly from the patient, without interpretation by a clinician or anyone else.

After an initial stage of not wanting to share her personal experience, Olivia now wishes to share it with other patients, health professionals, and the public. That is why she has started to write about her life as a patient (patient narrative; see subsection 2.3.6). She finds it useful – and even therapeutic – for herself and for society to share her personal narrative: her views, feelings and values.

2.3 Some current genres involving patients

Having reviewed the main theoretical issues related to genre and introduced Olivia, our character, we will now focus on the description of a selection of current genres involving genres as used in Western societies: patient information leaflets, fact sheets for patients, summaries for patients, informed consent forms, medical reports, patient reported outcomes and patient narratives.

2.3.1 The patient information leaflet

Every time we take medicine, whether it has been prescribed by the doctor or bought over the counter, we are provided with the relevant information about that medicine in a written document within the package called patient information leaflet – also referred to as PIL, information leaflet, package insert, patient package insert or consumer medicine information, depending on the context. Through this genre, pharmaceutical laboratories provide important information necessary for the correct use of medicines. Patient information leaflets are distributed by pharmaceutical manufacturers in one or more of three formats: package inserts, loose leaflets and electronic.

Many countries require this genre about drug therapy to be included in the medication package, and the content of this is mandated by regulatory guidelines. For example, in the European context, the patient information leaflet is required to ensure lay-friendly information "written and designed to be clear and understandable, enabling the users to act appropriately" (EU Directive 2001/83/EC). This text is structured in a particular order that patients expect and that reflects their needs for information in a logical sequence for that communicative situation; that is, taking the medicine in a safe and effective way.

1) What it is and what it is used for.
2) What you need to know before you start taking it.
3) How to take it.
4) Possible side effects.
5) Composition and contents of the pack.
6) Storage of the medicine.
7) Additional information.

FIGURE 2.2 Main sections of the patient information leaflet.

The first section deals with the identification of the medicine and its therapeutic indications. This part of the patient information leaflet provides the name, the active substance(s), the pharmaceutical form and the strength of the product. It informs the patient about all the substances with therapeutic activity (active ingredient), which are those that really act on our body, explaining the therapeutic group to which they belong and specifying the diseases that the medicine treats, describing the situations for which it is indicated based on previous scientific studies and approval by health authorities.

In this genre, we often find both non-proprietary names and commercial names of medicines. On the one hand, an international nonproprietary name (INN) identifies a pharmaceutical substance or active pharmaceutical ingredient by a unique name that is globally recognised and is public property. A nonproprietary name is also known as a generic name. The INN system was initiated in 1950 by the World Health Assembly to provide health professionals with a unique and universally available designated name to identify each pharmaceutical substance. On the other hand, the commercial name is key for patients to identify it correctly and ensure that they take the right medicine. Whereas INNs are internationally harmonised, commercial names can be problematic for translators because they often vary from language to language.

The second section typically offers information necessary to know before taking the medicine, such as contraindications, warnings and precautions regarding interactions with other medicines. This section also includes information on taking the medicine with certain food and drink, as well as information addressed to special groups of patients or general population, such as pregnant or nursing mothers.

The third section contains the most operational, user-centred type of information: the information that the patient as a reader will use to perform certain actions, such as taking the right amount of medicine at the right time and frequency. It also contains information about how long the course of treatment will last; what to do if a dose is missed; and if relevant, what do in the event of an overdose and the risk of withdrawal effects. The description of side effects is also highly relevant because it provides knowledge about what actions the patient should take if any of these occurred. The final sections are typically devoted to information about inactive ingredients details, a description of the product, registered pack sizes, storage conditions, and name and address of the manufacturer.

The World Health Organization (WHO) defines medication adherence as the degree that a person's behaviour corresponds with the agreed-on recommendations from a health care provider. Patient noncompliance with medicine leads to deterioration of illness, mortality and increased health care costs. One major factor that influences adherence is patients' ability to read and understand medication instructions. In addition to this, more than ever, consumers now want to know about their medicines and their impact to make informed choices. Survey findings tell us that patients want more information than they currently receive and that they value the patient information leaflet that comes with the medicine more highly than any other source of information except doctors and pharmacists (Medicines and Healthcare Products Regulatory Agency 2012).

However, patient information leaflets are not often lay-friendly (Jensen & Zethsen 2011), and patients struggle to understand them (Zethsen 2009; Maat & Lentz 2010), which can lead to lack of adherence and poor patient satisfaction. Thus, it is important to provide patients with informative, well set-out leaflets that are easy to navigate and that can lead to improved quality of life, reduce anxiety, promote early recognition of adverse side effects and provide a clear understanding of the treatment regimen. Chapters 5 and 6 in this book address comprehensibility and empathy issues in genres such as patient information leaflets. Good information helps patients participate fully in concordant decision-making about medicines prescribed for or recommended to them by health care professionals.

When translating or writing patient information leaflets, be aware that

- The text you create must guide the patient to take the medicine in a safe and effective way.
- In your context, there could be regulations regarding how to write patient information leaflets that you may need to consider.
- The commercial names of medicines vary from language to language.
- The instructions and explanations you provide must be clear and concise.
- Medical terminology must be presented in such a way that the patient understands it.

2.3.2 The fact sheet for patients

On many occasions, after leaving the consultation in which the doctor has provided us with the basic facts of a particular disease, we will have felt the need to know more about it. We do not always have the information to help us at hand. The fact sheet for patients - also referred to as patient brochure or information for patients - is aimed at patients who want or need to know more about a particular disease or condition. It is an informative genre that will help patients not only to better understand the relevant details of the disease but also to make decisions regarding treatment, manage symptoms, deal with disease processes, overcome periods of convalescence and adapt to a new lifestyle or adopt preventive measures. In contrast to patient information leaflets, fact sheets for patients do not have a fixed structure prescribed by law, but their structure and length vary according to the health care context and the institutions involved. It is a genre that is more institutionalised in Anglophone and European cultures than in other cultures. In fact, it is very common in the U.S. context, in which there is a long tradition in creating and translating – both inter-and intralingually – materials of all kinds for patients and making them available on the internet.

The sender or the writer of fact sheets for patients is usually a medical professional, an authoritative medical research body, a health association or a medical organisation that translates health information into easy-to-understand language and formats for patients to ensure their inclusion, education and empowerment. Ensuring inclusive access to information and communication often requires the use of multimodal solutions (see Chapter 3) that meet the specific needs of the target audience. An illustrative example is the Model Systems Knowledge Translation Center (https://msktc.org/), which provides a wide range of fact sheets for patients in a variety of formats, combining images with text for ease of access and understanding. However, all countries do not require that hospitals and health centres offer multilingual information, and in many cases this information is not available.

Regardless of the format and media, the fact sheet for patients is sometimes too formal for the literacy level of the readers being addressed; many patients do not know the basics of health, and the fact sheets can be deficient both in content (overly technical terminology or impersonal style) and in form (little use of images and unfriendly presentation), although the trend in recent times has been to increase the use of visual elements, especially with the proliferation of health sites on the internet. We are not referring to web-replicated genres, which have the same structure and information as printed genres and differ only in the means of access. We are referring to digital genres, which have the characteristics of web pages and offer the possibility of displaying information in a more attractive and interacting with the patient.

In the case of the printed paper format, there is also a gradual increase in the use of grammatical elements that aim to create a more personal bond with the readers (pronouns) and generate more empathy, such as using explanatory paraphrases or common collocations, shorter formats with questions and answers or drawings and images. In the digital formats, there is an attempt to adapt the contents to the different literacy levels of the target populations by producing different versions of the documents.

TASK 2.1 COMPARING FACT SHEETS FOR PATIENTS AND CONSIDERING THEIR ADEQUACY

Procedure

Compare these fact sheets for patients and discuss whether, in your opinion, the information they contain and the way it is conveyed is appropriate for an average health-literate audience in your context. Consider the complexity of the language, the use of unexplained terminology, the existence or not of images or other visual elements or their cultural appropriateness, the font type and colour(s), etc. Argue your answer.

Materials

1) Better Access to Mental Health Care. www1.health.gov.au/internet/main/publishing.nsf/Content/5DB6692978BC3395CA257BF0001C10D7/$File/factsheetforpatients.pdf
2) Know the facts About Coronavirus (Covid-19). https://familydoctor.org/know-the-facts-about-covid-19/
3) Health topics. www.who.int/health-topics/coronavirus#tab=tab_1

When translating or writing fact sheets for patients, be aware that

- The text you create must guide the patient to understand their clinical situation and adhere to treatment.
- You should address the patient in a direct and empathetic way.
- There must be coherence between the visual and the verbal elements.
- The information you provide must be clear and adequate.
- You should try to avoid using medical terms without explanations.

2.3.3 The summary for patients

The growing interest of patients and the public in learning about the latest medical investigations has increased the demand for texts that summarise research in ways they can understand. Increasingly, journals written by and for specialists now include simplified versions of research papers, which are reworded in the same language – that is, intra-lingually – to meet the needs of a lay readership. These versions are known as summaries for patients, a genre that to date is almost exclusively found in the biomedical field; these summaries written originally in languages other than English are scarce.

Summaries for patients are generally written either by researchers or by medical writers, although medical translators are sometimes called upon to produce these adaptations (Muñoz-Miquel 2014, 2016). Their overall social function is to democratise, and their purpose is to explain information about a specific study. They are aimed at lay readers who, as happens with readers of popular science magazines, may be interested in medicine or have a certain disease but have no medical background (see Chapter 4 for different types of readers).

Summaries for patients typically derive from original research articles. Original articles are highly conventionalised texts that aim to disseminate the results of rigorous research and convince the reader of its validity. This demand for accuracy requires the use of a fixed structure (IMRD: introduction, methods, results, discussion) and specialised terminology that is shared by the sender and the receiver, as both belong to the same community of specialists. Summaries for patients contain fewer technical terms and usually follow a question-and-answer structure, which runs parallel to that of the research article in that it helps to answer the questions posed in a research study. However, this structure is adapted to the new communicative situation and to the knowledge and expectations of the receiver. This question-and-answer structure contributes to the involvement of readers and builds a coherent picture of the facts that they are reading.

Figure 2.3 shows the structure of the original articles and the summaries for patients published by *Annals of Internal Medicine*, a biomedical journal that pioneered the creation of summaries from research articles (see http://annals.org/aim/pages/patient-information). The standard IMRD structure is transformed into questions and answers that respond to the same purposes as those of the sections of the original article but highly simplified.

When writing summaries for patients, the selection of the original content that is relevant to the patient is essential since this genre is meant to be much shorter than the original article. The writer explores the main ideas and chooses the most relevant, interesting and understandable ones for the new

Sections of the original article	Sections of the summary for patients	Purpose of the sections of the original article and the summary for patients
Introduction	What is the problem and what is known about it so far? Why did the researchers do this particular study?	– Define the problem. – Provide background information. – Show that the problem is interesting. – Establish hypotheses and objectives.
Methods	What was studied? How was the study done?	– Explain what was studied (participants, materials, etc.) and how (methods of analysis).
Results	What did the researchers find?	– Provide information about the results obtained.
Discussion	What were the limitations of the study? What are the implications of the study?	– Explain the results in the context of the study, the implications, the conclusions and the main limitations.

FIGURE 2.3 Typical structure of the original articles and the summaries for patients published in *Annals of Internal Medicine*.

Source: adapted from Muñoz-Miquel (2012).

reader. This requires having substantial knowledge of the original content, developing an ability to reason what must be kept and what can be left out and considering the readers' needs. For example, in general, patients are not interested in methods and statistics; that is, why the sections about methods are usually the shortest: statistical data and methodological details (participants inclusion and exclusion criteria, software to perform analyses, etc.) are deleted, and tables or figures are avoided. The emphasis is thus on the general results rather than the basic scientific and methodological details. However, it is important to strike a balance between relevance and accuracy because although patients do not need statistical information, they might be interested in the validity of the study (and this is usually reflected in the methods used).

Although summarising is crucial, relevant specific information about important concepts may need to be added or made explicit for a reader who does not have the same background knowledge about the subject matter as the writer. This type of more basic information is normally offered in the first section of the summary for patients. Regarding syntax and terminology, some strategies to make content more understandable and easier to read must be used, including making shorter sentences, using less jargon or providing examples (see Chapters 5 and 6).

Annals of Internal Medicine

Summary for Patients: Laparoscopic versus Open Surgery for Colorectal Liver Metastases

Author, Article, and Disclosure Information

What is the problem and what is known about it so far?

Most patients with metastatic colon or rectal cancer cannot be cured. However, a subset of such patients with isolated liver metastasis can have surgical removal, or resection, of the metastatic tumor in the liver, which might cure their disease. These patients have 2 surgical options for resection: an open or a laparoscopic approach.

Why did the researchers do this particular study?

To report the comparison of these 2 surgical approaches with respect to 5-year survival outcomes. The current study is the first randomized controlled trial comparing open versus laparoscopic resection of colorectal liver metastasis. The short-term results of this trial were already published and showed that the laparoscopic approach led to fewer complications within 30 days after surgery, faster recovery, and shorter hospital stay.

FIGURE 2.4 Extract of a summary for patients from *Annals of Internal Medicine* (www.acpjournals.org/doi/10.7326/P20–0012).

Not all summaries for patients derive from original articles. Some are produced based on clinical guidelines, used by health professionals in their clinical practice. The increasing need for user-friendly summaries has also led some medical organisations to publish summarised and simplified versions of symposiums to meet the information needs of specific groups of patients and their families. We can also find similar initiatives in some publications, such as medical treatises, which despite being aimed at medical professionals include summaries for patients, family members and caregivers (see, for example, *Understanding Liver Cancer*, Carr 2014). Summaries for patients should not be confused with full, non-summarised versions for patients (see the MSD Manual Consumer Version: www.msdmanuals.com/home).

TASK 2.2 EXPLORING TRANSFORMATION IN SUMMARIES FOR PATIENTS

Procedure

In the following links, you will find examples of summaries for patients from different genres: clinical guidelines, symposiums, original articles, evidence summaries, etc. Explore them and reflect on the changes that have been made to transform the specialised genres in summaries for patients.

Materials

1) *Annals of Internal Medicine*
   - Original article: www.acpjournals.org/doi/10.7326/m20-4011
   - Summary for patients: www.acpjournals.org/doi/10.7326/P20-0012
   - Clinical guideline: www.acpjournals.org/doi/10.7326/M15-2175
   - Summary for patients: www.acpjournals.org/doi/10.7326/P16-9016
2) National Institute of Allergy and Infectious Diseases
   - Clinical guideline www.niaid.nih.gov/diseases-conditions/guidelines-clinicians-and-patients-food-allergy
   - Summary for parents and caregivers: www.niaid.nih.gov/sites/default/files/peanut-allergy-prevention-guidelines-parent-summary.pdf
3) Aplastic Anemia & MDS International Foundation
   - Summary for patients from a symposium on the latest advances: www.aamds.org/sites/default/files/SymposiumPatientSummary.pdf

When translating or writing summaries for patients, be aware that

- The text must summarise an original article or a clinical guideline in a way that is relevant and understandable for a reader who may be interested in medicine or have a certain disease but is not a medical expert.
- You can follow a question–answer structure that responds to the main aspects of the text from which the summary derives.
- You should decide what the main ideas are and choose the most relevant considering the new reader's perspective.

- You should add or make explicit information about key concepts that need to be clarified for a reader with no medical background.
- Content, syntax and terminology must be easy to understand, so use shorter sentences and simpler terms or provide examples.

2.3.4 The informed consent

Every time a patient undergoes a diagnostic test, a surgical operation or a pharmacological treatment, in many health care systems, it is a medico-legal requirement for doctors to obtain the patient's consent. In the context of the informed consent, patients should be informed individually through direct dialogue with the doctor responsible for the procedure or treatment. This patient–doctor dialogue – in which patients express their concerns and ask questions about relevant issues, such as how the procedure is performed or the possible side effects it involves – leads to the signature of a written document: the informed consent form. This is a document typically containing all the relevant information about the procedure or treatment for the patient to make an informed decision about whether to consent to or decline it. The macrostructure of an informed consent form for a surgical operation is crucial to ensuring that patients have a comprehensive understanding of the procedure including its potential risks, benefits and alternatives before providing their consent. This information could vary depending on the health care system or the specific hospital. Figure 2.5 is a suggested macrostructure for an informed consent form for a surgical operation.

Title. Clearly states that the document is an informed consent form for a specific surgical operation.

Introduction. Briefly explains the purpose of the surgical procedure, emphasising the need for informed consent.

Patient information. Includes basic information about the patient, such as name, date of birth and medical record number.

Description of surgical procedure. Provides a detailed and understandable description of the surgical procedure, including the purpose, steps involved and any specific techniques or instruments that will be used.

Risks and complications. Clearly outlines potential risks and complications associated with the surgical operation. This section should cover both common and rare risks as well as the potential consequences of each.

Benefits. Describes potential benefits and outcomes of the surgical procedure, including improvements in health or relief of symptoms.

Alternative treatments. Explains any viable alternative treatments or procedures, including the risks and benefits associated with each. This helps patients make an informed decision about their health care.

Anaesthesia information. If the surgical procedure involves anaesthesia, this section provides information about the type of anaesthesia, potential risks and the role of the anaesthesiologist.

Voluntary participation. Emphasises that consenting to the surgical procedure is entirely voluntary and that the patient has the right to withdraw consent at any time without consequences.

Signature section. Provides a section for the patient to provide written consent by signing and dating the form. If applicable, a witness may also need to sign.

FIGURE 2.5 Macrostructure of an informed consent form for a surgical procedure.

By signing this document, the patient – or their legal representative in the case of children or patients unable to decide owing to a medical condition – authorises the doctor to perform or administer the proposed treatment or procedure. Informed consent is a performative speech act, the most explicit form being the patient's utterance, *I consent*. Patients have the right to accept or reject the proposed procedure or treatment, and this acceptance or rejection is communicated through an Informed consent form.

A patient's or participant's informed consent is also a medico-legal requirement in clinical trials. The macrostructure of this genre in the context of a clinical trial typically includes several key sections to ensure clarity and comprehensive information for the research participants. Figure 2.6 is a suggested macrostructure for an informed consent form for participating in a research study.

Both in clinical trials and in health care, participants and patients must be informed individually in addition to receiving the informed consent form in a written document. In Western societies, consent to medical care is a fundamental ethical practice because it is the way patients autonomously authorise medical interventions or courses of treatment. This prerogative to

Title. Clearly states that the document is an informed consent form for a specific research study.

Introduction. Briefly explains the purpose of the study and provides an overview of what the participant will be asked to do.

Study information. Details the background and objectives of the research, including the research question or hypothesis.

Procedures. Describes the specific procedures involved in the study, including any interventions or treatments, the duration of the study and the frequency and nature of participant involvement.

Risks and benefits. Clearly outlines potential risks and benefits associated with participation in the study. This section may also include information about any alternative treatments or procedures.

Confidentiality. Explains how participant confidentiality will be maintained and the steps taken to protect their privacy.

Voluntary participation. Emphasises that participation in the study is entirely voluntary and that the participant has the right to withdraw at any time without consequences.

Contact information. Provides contact details for the researchers, including principal investigators and key personnel, so participants can ask questions or seek additional information.

Participant rights. Outlines the rights of the participant, including the right to ask questions, the right to be informed of any new information that may affect their willingness to continue and the right to withdraw from the study.

Signature section. Includes spaces for the participant to provide written consent by signing and dating the form. For studies involving minors, a parent or legal guardian may also need to sign.

Witness signature. In some cases, a witness (someone who is not involved in the study) may be required to sign the form, confirming that the participant voluntarily consented and was adequately informed.

FIGURE 2.6 Macrostructure of an informed consent form in a clinical trial.

control one's medical destiny is elemental (Joffe & Truog 2010). There are five aspects that establish the conditions for valid consent in doctor–patient relationships in standard clinical settings (Figure 2.7).

A crucial ethical aspect of informed consent is patients' adequate understanding (see Chapter 5). Disclosure is not enough; uninformed and ill-informed patients, and patients who are unfamiliar with the language, cannot consent in a valid way. To achieve a sufficient degree of understanding on the part of the patient requires the appropriate register, that is, a text written in adequate detail and in a language that is familiar to the patient (Kleinig 2010: 16).

In theory, informed consent should not only have medico-legal validity, it should also be truly meaningful to the patient. In the practice of writing and translation of consent forms, the medico-legal dimension, and often its defensive role, take centre stage, and the ethical, cognitive and affective dimensions tend to vanish. In many health care contexts, signing a consent form is a mere formality prior to surgery or tests. Informed consent should constrain the power of physicians; this is something that patients seldom realise. Most of these documents tend to lack transparency, contain too much technical terminology, and are depersonalised, focusing on the medical dimension and leaving aside the emotional dimension (Montalt 2022). To overcome these limitations, there are several initiatives such as the i-Consent project (https://i-consentproject.eu/) or the Hipocrates project by the GENTT group (https://hipocratesgentt.uji.es/) – meant to improve both the process and the written document of this genre.

1) The patient must be free to make a decision without feeling under pressure.
2) The patient must be competent (i.e. with full consciousness and cognitive abilities).
3) The patient must be made aware of the relevant facts, such as the nature and purpose of any procedure, its risks and potential benefits and any alternative options.
4) The patient must be able to demonstrate full understanding of the disclosed facts.
5) The patient must either authorise or decline the proposed course of treatment.

FIGURE 2.7 Conditions for valid consent in doctor–patient relationships.

In the context of this genre, the relationship between patient and health professional is fiduciary in nature; a fiduciary is a person entrusted for the benefit of another and legally held to the highest standard of conduct. Fiduciaries advise and represent others and manage their affairs. In this regard, the role of translators and interpreters can also be seen as that of a fiduciary entrusted to act in interlingual and intercultural communication on behalf of both the patient and the health professional. Consequently, informed consent poses some relevant questions for interpreters and translators, such as whether the translator or interpreter should promote awareness of it or should contribute and ensure that it is fulfilled ethically.

When translating or writing informed consents, be aware that

- Patients who read informed consent forms are involved in a crucial process of decision-making regarding their health.
- Informed consent is an individual act that involves a dialogue between the patient and the health professional before the patient finally gives or declines consent.
- Patients should be informed ethically, which involves both adequate medical content and adequate linguistic and textual form. this is crucial for them to decide whether to give consent and authorise a procedure or course of treatment.
- Register should be adequate for patients, regardless of the register inadequacies found in the source text.
- Ensuring comprehensibility is paramount. If patients do not understand the consent form, then they will sign it blindly, which is unethical.

2.3.5 The medical report

Who has never been to an emergency department or to a medical consultation either to be treated or to take a relative or a friend? In some countries, at the end of the visit, we are given a report explaining the reasons why we went to the clinic, the diagnosis we received and the treatment that was prescribed. We are usually told to keep this discharge report and give it to our general practitioner.

During our visit, the doctor might have explained to us orally what is wrong and what treatment we should follow. However, once we get home, we may realise that there are details – for example, how we should take the medicine prescribed – that we do not remember. This makes us read the report carefully to search for more information. More often than not, we notice that we are facing a document written in our language and talking about our health that we do not completely understand: it is generally jargon-ridden and full of terms, abbreviations or symbols we are unfamiliar with. Why does this happen? What is this document for? Who is its target audience?

This report is known as a medical report or health report. It is a document in which the doctor who is taking care of a patient – or the attending physician in a certain episode of care – shares the patient's medical condition, including diagnosis, examinations, treatments and so on. It serves as a record of a patient's health condition. The medical report, which can be of many types (discharge summary, consultation report, pathology report, among others) is part of the medical record (also referred to as medical history, not to be confused with a medical report), which, as seen in subsection 2.1.1, serves to collect all of a person's medical information. The main objective of a medical report (and of a medical record) is to provide health care professionals who may treat a patient at any time with complete information concerning the patient's health. Then, medical reports help communication among doctors.

However, patients have also access to their medical reports despite not being their primary recipients (see the concept of *overhearer* in Chapter 4), and these reports can enhance their knowledge about their health. Other functions of these reports include providing data that help researchers perform epidemiological, public health, and other related investigations; supporting the theoretical and practical teaching of medicine and serving as a record of the care provided to a patient in the event of complaints or legal proceedings on the medical procedures performed (Da Costa 1996; Delàs 2005; NHS Digital 2018).

Unlike other genres that are clearly and only addressed to patients and relatives that we have explained in previous sections (patient information leaflets, fact sheets for patients, informed consent forms), the medical report addresses a varied audience (Estopà 2020; Domènech-Bagaria et al. 2020): medical professionals, patients and their relatives, researchers and documentalists, lecturers and students of medicine, even jurists (see Chapter 4). These receivers do not share the same knowledge, have different concerns about the text (Estopà & Domènech-Bagaria 2019) and will use it in different ways. This variation explains how difficult it is to write a text that fits everyone's needs and expectations. Figure 2.8 is a suggested macrostructure for a patient medical report (Delàs 2005; Llopart-Saumel & Da Cunha 2020).

From a linguistic point of view, some of the characteristics of a medical report include the following:

- Very concise and depersonalised writing style
- Predominance of the passive voice

- Patient identification data (name, medical record number, date of birth, gender, etc.)
- Presenting complaint or reason for admission (reasons and symptoms that caused a patient to seek medical care)
- Past medical history (allergies, chronic diseases, previous illnesses, surgical interventions, family history if relevant, etc.)
- Physical exam and investigations (general and body systems review, investigations and tests performed, examinations findings, etc.)
- Diagnosis
- Treatments and interventions (pharmacological, surgical, etc.)
- Clinical course and follow-up (description of how the disease behaves over time)
- Date and signature of the attending practitioner

FIGURE 2.8 Macrostructure of a medical report.

- High terminological density
- Extensive use of acronyms, abbreviations, and symbols that are not clarified (Delàs 2005; Hansen & Zethsen 2018; Domènech-Bagaria et al. 2020; Estopà & Montané 2020).

These characteristics usually make it difficult for those who do not have a medical background – patients and their relatives – to understand medical reports. Medical professionals often write these reports without considering that patients could also be potential receivers (not just overhearers, see Chapter 4) and have the right to fully understand them.

In addition, health professionals usually find it difficult to write about their field in a way lay people can understand it (expert blind spot), which makes the problem worse. This fact can lead to poor adherence to treatments, increased convalescence time, self-diagnosis owing to uncritical searchers for medical information on the internet and communication gaps that increase inequality between patients and health care professionals. Therefore, there is a lot of room for improvement related to writing medical reports in a more comprehensible way without compromising accuracy (see more about barriers to understanding in Chapter 5).

However, it is not all about patients' understanding. Comprehension problems can also affect other users of the medical report – medical professionals, documentalists, researchers, and so on. Aleixandre-Benavent et al. (2006) showed that many of the abbreviations found in medical reports are invented by the author, are not agreed upon by the medical community or have different meanings depending on the context. This makes them difficult to understand by experts, too.

Suggestions for task. Medical reports

To what extent do you think medical reports can be made comprehensible, taking into account that patients are not the only (or the primary target readers) of these reports? Discuss your views on this with a colleague.

In today's eHealth scenarios, writing understandable reports is especially relevant. Most medical records are now found in electronic format (e-record) to facilitate interoperability and easy access to health information. To promote patient-centredness and patient empowerment, there are countries in which e-records are easily accessible by patients in only a few clicks; see Hansen and Zethsen (2018) for a description of the situation in Denmark. However, the problem remains the same: although these records are supposed to function as patient information, they can only be understood by experts. See Figure 2.9 for an example.

Clinical synthesis

87-year-old patient treated with long-term (since 2016) parenteral iron replacement and repeated erythrocyte transfusions. However, at the beginning of March 2018, a drop of Hb of almost 40 g/l in less than 3 weeks was detected, therefore admitted to our clinic for blood transfusions and investigation of the etiology of the losses.

Gastrofibroscopy without evidence of bleeding, colonoscopy showed blood in the colon, but the source was not found, presumably in the small intestine.

Source of bleeding was not detected even by double balloon enteroscopy and repeat capsule enteroscopy (2022). In the following period, the hemoglobin value was above 100 g/L with a few exceptions.

Now electively admitted for an endoscopic examination of the terminal ileum by colonoscopy, which revealed angiectasias in the ascending colon (apparently covered by blood in the earlier acute colonoscopy) and a small polyp of the sigmoid colon (biopsy taken). After discontinuation of anticoagulant therapy, transient ischemic attack with left-sided hemiparesis occurred on May 11, 2022, which resolved spontaneously during transfer for brain CT scan.

Therefore, she was secured with heparin and switched to the lowest still effective dose of direct anticoagulant. Subsequently, destruction by argon plasmacoagulation via colonoscopy was performed without complications. Prior to dimission, i.v. iron was administered.

FIGURE 2.9 Extract from a discharge report published in the Guidelines on Hospital Discharge Report, Release 1, Nov. 2023, adopted by the eHealth Network (https://health.ec.europa.eu/system/files/2024–01/ehn_hdr_guidelines_en.pdf).

When translating or writing medical reports, be aware that

- The medical report is part of the medical record or medical history.
- Unlike other genres, a medical report addresses a very varied audience – medical professionals, patients, researchers, documentalists, medical students, and so on – who will use it in different ways.
- This variety of receivers poses great challenges for translators, as it is very difficult to write a report that fits everyone's needs and expectations.
- Medical reports are generally only understandable by experts, but you should consider that patients are also proper receivers and must fully understand them.
- Writing understandable reports is especially relevant if they are in electronic format (e-record), as they are more easily accessible by patients. This can promote patient-centredness and patient empowerment.

2.3.6 The patient reported outcome

When we take a medicine or when some kind of health policy is activated in a particular context or country (for example, vaccinations), a complex process of expert decision-making that often involves patients has normally preceded them. In these processes, feasibility studies are crucial. They are performed to gather and analyse the opinions and perceptions of those involved (i.e. patients and health professionals) to make informed decisions that will be effective for the purpose in hand.

In the context of clinical research, clinical outcome assessments are measures that reflect a patient's health condition and are used in clinical trials to assess the effectiveness of new treatments. This information about the patient can be obtained from different sources: a doctor, an observer (such as a caregiver or a relative) or the patient himself. The patient reported outcome (also called PRO) is a type of clinical outcome assessment reported by the patients themselves in which they provide information about their health condition without outside interpretation from anyone. This is a genre that originated in English-speaking medical contexts, such as the US Food and Drug Administration, but that is translated into multiple languages owing to the interests of potential clients (organisations, clinical centres, research groups and, primarily, the pharmaceutical industry) in different countries.

Several tools (called patient reported outcome measures or PROMs) are used for patients to report on a wide variety of health relevant aspects, such as:

- Health-related quality of life (HRQoL), which refers to an individual's subjective perception and evaluation of their physical health, mental well-being and overall quality of life related to their health status. It can be generic or condition specific.

- Functional status, which reflects the ability to perform specific activities (e.g. driving).
- Symptoms and symptom burden, which focus on types of symptoms of interest that may have not been captured by doctors in the consultation.
- Health behaviours, which refer to the self-reported actions or activities that individuals engage in that directly impact their health status or HRQoL.
- Patient experience, which concerns satisfaction with health care delivery, treatment recommendations and medications (or other therapies). It reflects actual experiences with health care services and fosters patient activation (Cella et al. 2015).

The people who prepare patient reported outcome measures are usually doctors and their teams or sponsoring organisations, but translation agencies and their translators, who also act as auditors, play a vital role in the process of gathering information from patients in a specific language and country. With the results obtained from all the evaluation tests, decisions can be made on important aspects such as health policies or on the acceptability of a medicine. This is a genre in which the role of the translator as mediator is fundamental, especially because of the implications that translation can have in health systems and cultures different from English-speaking countries, not only in linguistic terms but also regarding the cultural interpretation of the relevant information.

Patient reported outcomes tend to be country and culture specific; their reports carry with them embedded linguistic and cultural nuances. Thus, cross-cultural adaptation is relevant in this genre because different cultures and languages can have unique expressions, meanings and concepts related to health, illness and quality of life. The goal of effective translation and cross-cultural adaptation is therefore to acknowledge these features to provide a reliable and valid alternative for the target language and/or culture and ensure equivalence between the source and the target versions of patient reported outcomes.

Unlike genres such as the informed consent or the fact sheet for patients, which provide information to the patient, patient reported outcomes are characterised by the exact opposite: they extract information from the patient. In contrast to the patient narrative, the purpose of the this genre is not to express the subjective experience of patients' illness but to extract from the patient those data that are relevant to the strategy of a company or health care organisation in feasibility studies of certain products or services.

When dealing with patient reported outcomes, be aware that

- You need to carry out cultural adaptation regarding health and illness.
- You need to address the patient in a clear way and to avoid using medical terminology without an explanation.
- You need to ensure that you have clearly understood the patient and every part of what they have reported.

2.3.7 The patient narrative

Narratives pervade health care. Narrative medicine has been proposed as a model for humane and effective medical practice that draws on the power of verbal accounts of genuine human experience (Charon 2001). Proponents suggest that the patient–doctor relationship can be improved by encouraging a form of interaction in which both parties engage in more narrative and balanced ways in terms of power and status. Narrative medicine is based on the notions of active listening to patients' narratives, emotional and cultural alignment with their experiences and careful attention to non-biomedical aspects of health.

In the consultation, patients tell their stories to doctors. The anamnesis – originally meaning the ability to recall past events – begins with a chief complaint presented by the patient in the consultation. It continues with a history of the current illness and the medical, surgical and family history and ends with an assessment, possibly a diagnosis and a therapeutic plan. The sequence of events and experiences narrated by the patient, encouraged by the doctor to provide relevant information, forms the basis for the written case history. From these oral accounts, doctors write a medical case history: the written account of the patient's illness.

The fundamental tenet of narrative medicine is that meaning is constructed in the stories that we tell. In medicine, many stories are told. Patients tell stories about symptoms, illnesses or concerns; their contexts; how they are being affected and why they came to see the doctor. These stories have infinite variations in content, the people telling them, the languages they use and the ways they tell their stories. Narratives reflect the uniqueness of individual patients and their personal experiences.

Doctors also bring their own stories to the consultation. The doctor's understanding of what is occurring to the patient, the diagnosis that is made and the ideas about causes and management form a story that must be communicated to the patient. The way in which this is conducted reflects the doctor's personality, knowledge, cultural awareness, listening skills, experiences and practice.

Narratives can have different uses. In the context of clinical trials, narratives often consist of brief summaries of the adverse effects that patients experience when taking a particular drug. These narratives are typically attached to the clinical trial report in the form of an appendix and submitted to regulatory authorities. They are written by medical writers, and their purpose is to help to determine the safety profile of the drug under study. Although automation (i.e. machine-generated writing) of narrative is an emerging trend in the pharmaceutical sector as it provides quality and consistency, human review is always a must to ensure that it makes sense.

So far, we have referred to narrative medicine as it is used in consultations and in clinical trials. Now we will shift our attention to how patients write their own narratives beyond clinical settings and become active agents in the communication process. In recent years, patients are increasingly feeling the need to share their experiences of illness beyond their family and friends. Patients tell their personal experiences to other patients and to any reader or viewer/listener eager to know about them, including health professionals, and they become visible in the public arena – through social networks, blogs, interviews or even more formal publications such as books.

The internet offers many possibilities for digital storytelling. Web-based patient narratives have become widely available on the internet and social media. These narratives have a high potential to add unknown insights into patient-focused issues that can only be provided by someone who has gone through a similar experience. In their stories, patients use a variety of narrative devices to express their personal experiences of illness. They could refer to past events in clinical contexts and to their encounters with doctors from whom they have learned new medical concepts.

To express their experiences, patients can use medical terminology that they have learned through their interactions with health professionals. They can also focus on more subjective issues related to their feelings and the way they perceive the process they are going through. For example, in patients' narratives, we find metaphorical expressions (Semino & Demjén 2017; Vandaele 2018) such as *the war against disease* or *illness is a journey*. Metaphor is well known to be a linguistic and cognitive tool that we use to think and talk about subjective, sensitive and complex experiences in terms of experiences that tend to be simpler and more intersubjectively accessible. Illness is an experience that is often talked about and conceptualised through metaphor (Semino 2020, 2021). Metaphors can empower or disempower patients, and there is a backlash in the literature about the sometimes dehumanising effect of illness as a metaphor (e.g. Susan Sontag's 1978 essay *Illness as Metaphor*).

Patient Voices (www.patientvoices.org.uk) is just one of the many projects in which you can find examples of patients becoming storytellers who share their personal experiences through written text or videos. Reflective digital storytelling of this kind can be useful not only to patients but also to health professionals and students. Patient narratives can fulfil several functions in the health system and in society at large. They can support other patients experiencing similar problems and challenges in coping with their illness. They can also serve as a resource for exploring and making health care decisions. For example, they can help to identify information and communication problems. Finally, they can point to new clinical issues for physicians. For some researchers, the concern is that patients' decision-making regarding treatment options could be based on the personal experiences of the few, whereas statistical data remain largely ignored (Drewniak et al. 2020).

TASK 2.3 BECOMING AWARE OF PATIENTS' EXPERIENCES OF ILLNESS

Part 1

Procedure and materials

1) Read the following editorial from the BMJ, "The transformative power of patient narratives in healthcare education" (https://blogs.bmj.com/bmj/2019/07/08/the-transformative-power-of-patient-narratives-in-healthcare-education/)
2) The authors of this opinion state that "patient voices should be equal to those of others involved in the education and regulation of healthcare professionals".

   - Do you think that patients should be involved actively in educational and regulatory issues regarding health care? Why?
   - What power do patient voices have when expressed in their own unaltered forms and languages?
   - What is the patients' form and language in your culture?

Part 2

Procedure and materials

1) Google "patient stories" or "patient narratives" (or similar expressions) in your target language and choose a few of them. They can be written text or videos, or even podcasts.
2) Read – or watch/listen to – them and explore the following issues: What structural pattern do they follow? What types of information do they contain? What do you think is the purpose of their authors? How can other patients and health professionals benefit from such narratives?
3) Watch this seminar for a full understanding of metaphor: http://repositori.uji.es/xmlui/handle/10234/191538?show=full
4) Now focus on the metaphors patients use in the narratives you found. In which metaphorical terms do they talk about their experiences? Do they use war metaphors? Or perhaps they prefer travel or other metaphors? Which other metaphors do they use?
5) Finally, if your target language is not English, google similar patient narratives in English and compare the ways English-speaking patients express their experiences with the preferences shown by the patients in your target language. How long are the narratives in both languages? Are they structured in the same way? Do they contain the same type of information? Do they use the same types of metaphors? How do they differ?

When translating or writing patient narratives, be aware that

- The language used by patients in their narratives is very valuable because it reflects their experiences and can provide important clues in the understanding of individual illness.
- Patients' language reflects social, cultural and individual aspects.
- The emotional dimension is a fundamental part of patients' narratives.
- Formally speaking, patients' narratives can vary notably not only between languages and cultures but also within the same language and culture.
- Writing and translating individuality and self-perception pose different challenges than translating biomedical discourse.

2.4 Emerging genres involving patients

We conclude this chapter with the presentation of health apps and comics as examples of emerging genres in which multimodal approaches (see Chapter 3) to patient-centred communication, writing and translation are crucial.

2.4.1 The health app

Most of us cannot image our lives without a smartphone. Besides making phone calls and texting, we use smartphones to browse the internet, take pictures, receive directions through GPS, play games, keep track of appointments and contacts and so on. The spread of mobile technologies has had a major impact on the health care field. Mobile health technology is the use of smartphones, tablets, and other mobile devices and wearables to improve health care delivery, access and research (Singh & Landman 2017). Mobile health has evolved as a field of eHealth, which is the use of information and communication technologies for health (WHO 2022).

Imagine the following scenarios:

- A patient receives a text message reminding her of her upcoming gynaecological visit. She confirms her appointment and asks her smartphone to remind her one hour before her visit.
- A patient sends an email to her daughter's doctor with a picture of a rash because she does not know if she has to be seen in the doctor's office or if the rash can be treated with an over-the-counter medicine. Telemedicine allows her to speak with her child's doctor from the comfort of her own home.
- A teenaged diabetes patient uses an app on her smartphone to enter her glucose readings, earning points for readings within the desired range. She uses the same app to play games that reinforce ways she can help manage her diabetes with her diet.

What do all these scenarios have in common? They are all examples of how mobile health can help patients easily monitor their health, establish closer contact with health care providers and participate more actively in their care. The role of apps is becoming especially relevant, and they can yield many benefits. In fact, there are international initiatives and best practices (eHealth Action Plan 2012–2020 by the European Union or the WHO Global Strategy on Digital Health) that promote the adoption and spread of mobile health among consumers, health care providers, and health care systems.

Mobile health apps are usually created and developed by private medical companies and software and app developers (e.g. AthenaHealth, CareCloud, ScienceSoft). There is a wide range of apps that register users' different health biometrics (heart rate, blood sugar levels, sleep, etc.); encourage the user to change unhealthy habits (e.g. smoking); help doctors support clinical decisions and keep up with medical news, new drug releases, medicines and their effects and are used by health authorities to track public health issues.

Mobile health apps can be aimed at medical professionals and health care providers or intended for use by patients and consumers in general. Those intended for health care providers help them access clinical information, monitor patients in real time, provide emergency response and collaborate with care teams among other features. Epocrates® is an example of a provider-facing app; most patient-facing apps are fitness, well-being and diet based, but some are used for chronic disease management (e.g. apps to monitor blood glucose levels among diabetics). Apps aimed at chronic disease patients allow them to view their health within a narrative context as patients create and see the story of their own health.

2.4.2 The comic

Many people enjoy reading comic strips, especially children, and most associate this genre with entertainment. It is a traditional genre that has not been widely used for health promotion until recently. The intersection between the medium of comics and the discourse of health care has been coined graphic medicine, in which the image sequence format of cartoons and comics has started to be used to tell health-related stories and generate a response in the reader.

The basic objective in the use of comic strips in patient-centred communication is health promotion, education, prevention and improvement of the quality of life of patients and their relatives. This genre is also used as an educational tool in training health professionals. Comics have the advantage of being an attractive genre to the reader and presenting information in a brief, easy-to-understand way. They combine the explicit meaning of words and symbols with the abstract expressiveness of visual art.

Despite its pervasive presence, comics are a rather complex genre; they have different names – cartoons, graphic novels, comic strips – as well as different purposes. They address different audiences, including children or adolescents, but also adults. In comics we find different registers depending on the target audience and the purpose. Formats can also vary, including vignettes of many types – in colour or in black and white and with different fonts – and both as an independent medium or inserted as part of a periodical publication.

The sender of the comic can be a public organisation, such as a hospital, a health centre or even an individual health professional, or a private one such as patients' associations or companies in the medical and health sectors. Sometimes this genre is used by individual patients to express a personal experience of illness in a brief and attractive way.

Comics have the particularity of combining verbal (which is usually included in the balloons to convey the thoughts of the characters and in the captions for the narrator) and non-verbal, which gives significance to its discourse (onomatopoeias, visual metaphors or the use of perspective, which according to some studies gives it a certain emotional dimension) language. This multimodal discourse allows the writer or translator to project content beyond the purely medical to include the social, psychological and cultural aspects surrounding disease and illness that are specific to different cultures and social groups. For further information about graphic medicine, please explore graphicmedicine.org, a community of academics, health professionals, authors, artists and fans of comics and medicine.

Suggestions for task. Discovering the comic as a patient-centred genre

Discuss the following questions with your classmates or colleagues: Do you know any comics about health? Do you think it is a common genre in your culture? In what context and for what type of population would you use this genre on a regular basis?

There is a wealth of patient-centred genres that writers and translators must be familiar with. This great diversity reflects the richness that characterises patient-centred communication and can contribute conceptual and methodological orientations for the analysis and production of texts. Using genres can facilitate patient-centred communication in multilingual and multicultural health care settings for several reasons.

First, genres enable us to develop a more situated approach in which participants and their intentions, expectations and needs take centre stage. Second, genres enable us to understand structural, conceptual, pragmatic and stylistic diversity and variability when addressing patients. Third, they help us anticipate writing and translating problems in specific communicative situations; in particular, they help us establish hierarchies regarding the most salient aspect of each genre – including structure, types of information, register or ethical orientation of the overall communicative event – that can guide the production of the target text.

However, genres addressing or involving patients also pose challenges in the practical arena. They don't always respond to patients' needs and expectations; that is, they are not always patient centred. Thus, in many cases, imitating and replicating in our target texts the characteristics of the texts that we find in real situations may not be the best approach. Ensuring patient-centred language quality in the texts we produce requires critical thinking and the development of analytical and production skills regarding multimodality (Chapter 3), audience analysis (Chapter 4), comprehensibility (Chapter 5) and empathy (Chapter 6).

Further reading

Alkureishi, M. A., et al. Impact of an Educational Comic to Enhance Patient-Physician–Electronic Health Record Engagement: Prospective Observational Study. *JMIR Human Factors*, 2021, *8* (2), e25054.

Bhatia, V. Applied Genre Analysis: A Multi-Perspective Model. *Ibérica: Revista de la Asociación Europea de Lenguas para fines específicos (AELFE)*, 2002, 4, 3–19.

García-Izquierdo, I., Ed. *El género textual y la traducción: reflexiones teóricas y aplicaciones pedagógicas*; Peter Lang: Berna, 2005.

García-Izquierdo, I. *Divulgación médica y traducción: el género información para pacientes*; Peter Lang: Berna, 2009.

Jensen, M. N. *Translators of Patient Information Leaflets: Translation Experts or Expert Translators? A Mixed Methods Study of Lay-Friendliness*; Department of Business Communication: Aarhus University, 2013.

Montalt, V. Ethical Considerations in the Translation of Health Genres in Crisis Communication. In *Translating Crises*; O'Brien, S.; Federici, F. M., Eds.; Bloomsbury Publishing, 2022, p. 17.

Pilegaard, M.; Ravn, H. B. Readability of Patient Information Can Be Improved. *Danish Medical Journal*, 2012, *59* (5), A4408.

Pilegaard, M. The Ethics of Informed Consent: An Applied Linguistics Perspective. In *Medical Discourse in Professional, Academic and Popular Settings*; Multilingual Matters, 2016; 79–102.

Semino, E.; Demjén, Z., Eds. *The Routledge Handbook of Metaphor and Language*; Routledge Handbooks in Linguistics; Routledge: London; New York, 2017.

Shuttleworth, M. *Studying Scientific Metaphor in Translation: An Inquiry Into Cross-Lingual Translation Practices*; Routledge Advances in Translation and Interpreting Studies; Routledge: New York; London, 2017.

Sontag, S. *Illness as Metaphor and AIDS and Its Metaphors*; Macmillan, 2001.

Tvedten, O., et al. Personalised Written Consultation Summaries for Patients: An 'Up-Close, in-Depth, Inside-Out' Exploration of a Rheumatologist's Patient-Centred Strategy. *Patient Education and Counseling*, 2022, *105* (7), 2362–2370.

3

EXPLORING MULTIPLE MODES, CODES, FORMATS AND MEDIA

Overview of chapter

Although this book is concerned primarily with different kinds of written communication, it is important to understand that written material may also be used in oral and audio-visual settings. This chapter focuses on the existence of and the interplay between multiple modes (oral, written, audio-visual), codes (verbal and non-verbal), formats (layout, typography) and media (printed documents, webs pages, apps and other digital technologies) – which we refer to as *multimodality* – that can be used to cater to specific needs in effective and inclusive communication. This chapter covers three main areas.

After we define what the concept of multimodality entails (Section 3.1), the first area we address is the medical consultation, the central oral genre in patient–doctor communication (Section 3.2). In any conversation, there is what is said but also body language, which sometimes can communicate more than words. In the face-to-face consultation, both verbal and non-verbal (eye contact or use of physical space) languages are used in a wide range of ways and situations, from communicating minor issues to breaking bad news. Although the consultation (both when it is mediated by an interpreter and when it is not mediated) is based on spoken interaction, it can often involve information in the form of images and texts.

Face-to-face consultations are gradually giving way to remote consultations by email, telephone or videoconferencing, which pose new multimodal challenges. To improve the interaction between the patient and the doctor, good practice guidelines are useful, but they are not used or even not available at all in all countries. Roleplays can also be helpful for improving communication through the training of health professionals and interpreters in communication skills.

DOI: 10.4324/9780429299698-4

The second area deals with the needs of patients who are blind or partially sighted, deaf or hard of hearing or have learning difficulties (Section 3.3). As a consequence, they don't have direct access to standard information and communication in health care and are at risk of being left out. The focus is then on accessibility and inclusivity. Writers, translators and interpreters must be aware of these special needs. Audio descriptions of images for the blind and sign language and subtitles in videos for the deaf and hard of hearing can be used when addressing such audiences. Adapting information and communication to the circumstances and needs of patients with learning difficulties through the use of images and simplified language is another aspect to be considered.

The third area focuses on the new ways of delivering health care in the era of mobile communications and the internet (Section 3.4). The digital patient is on the way. New apps, blogs, websites and other digital resources and media are being developed to cater for the fast-changing needs of the digital patient, whose presence online is becoming ever more prominent. There are all sorts of health apps to assist patients. Electronic health is even more on the rise in the times of Covid-19.

3.1 Approaching multimodality

Together with the text, the register, the code, the linguistic system and the social structure (Halliday 1995), the situation (see Chapter 2) is an essential component of the sociosemiotic theory of language that underpins our approach to patient-centred translation and communication in this book. The situation is the environment in which the text comes to life, and it can be represented as a complex of three dimensions: the ongoing social activity (field), the role relationship involved (tenor) and the symbolic or rhetorical channel (mode) (Halliday 1995). The mode is thus the channel or wavelength chosen and includes the medium, traditionally spoken and written but now also audio-visual.

Based on Halliday's functional systemic linguistics, multimodality is a concept that has been introduced and developed over the last three decades to account for the different resources used in communication to express meaning (Adami 2017). The term is used both to describe a phenomenon of human communication and to identify a diverse and growing field of research (Adami 2017). Within the field of multimodal studies (O'Halloran & Smith 2012), four key assumptions seem to dominate: 1) all communication is multimodal; 2) an analysis that focuses solely or primarily on verbal language cannot adequately account for meaning; 3) each mode has specific affordances that arise from its materiality and social history; 4) modes work together, each with a specialised role, to make meaning; therefore, the relationships between modes are key to understanding any instance of communication and contributing to its improvement.

Jakobson's (1959) distinction between intralingual, interlingual and intersemiotic translation is a good example of the long-standing interest in multimodality in translation studies. Intersemiotic translation is "an interpretation of verbal signs by means of signs of non-verbal sign systems" (Jakobson 1959: 233). Over the years, and with radical technological developments, this earlier theoretical concern with multimodality has evolved into more practical questions that are relevant to this chapter, such as whether the same concept can be best expressed by a verbal sign or text in one language or culture and by an image in another, or what the translator's responsibilities in this kind of situations are, or how the translator should take into account multiple semiotic resources to address diverse audiences (Rike 2013).

3.2 Multimodality in the medical consultation

During her therapeutic process as a patient, Olivia has gone through different stages and has needed different types of information provided through different formats and media beyond the oral consultation itself. Sometimes she has been given printed materials, but she has also visited web pages that health professionals or other patients recommended and even used mobile apps.

The interaction between doctor and patient in the clinical context takes place mainly in the medical consultation. Depending on the linguistic needs of either the patient or the doctor, or both, it may have to be mediated by an interpreter. The medical consultation has a central function in healthcare since it is in this communicative event or genre that a more personalised and direct relationship can be establish. The medical consultation is the basic tool of health care and, like health care itself, it has evolved and continues to evolve over time. In consultations, patients provide information that enable doctors to reach diagnoses and in turn receive information that hopefully enables them to understand and comply with the therapeutic process.

Face-to-face consultations, where verbal and non-verbal information can be shared, have many advantages. The first and most obvious one is self-identification of both the patient and the doctor. In addition, a patient can convey meanings not only through words but also through eye contact and gestures, such as pointing to a specific part of the body or communicating by facial expressions. Furthermore, a doctor can gather all sorts of information about patients' concerns by combining verbal and physical means.

Many genres are predominantly either oral, such as a conference lecture or written, like a patient information leaflet. However, in other genres, such as the medical consultation, the boundaries between the oral and the written modes are not always clear-cut and depend on multiple factors, including the needs and preferences of the patients and what actually occurs in a given interaction.

3.2.1 Visual and written resources in the consultation

Although the medical consultation is basically an oral interaction, it may nevertheless make use of written language if needed, either in the consultation itself or beyond it. Images can be used as meaningful visual representations of concepts which complement a text or a conversation. It has been shown that they make it easier for patients to grasp specialised concepts that would otherwise require more detailed verbal explanation (Prieto & Montalt 2018).

There can be multiple reasons to use visual information. For example, the doctor may use pictures, infographics or diagrams to explain a surgical procedure or the cause of a medical condition or to indicate types of exercises that would help patients to strengthen muscles after surgery. They may also be used to help the doctor to give clear explanations to children, the elderly, patients with learning difficulties and people with low literacy. In addition, empowered and proactive patients like Olivia may require additional, more detailed information beyond that provided orally in the consultation.

Both patients and doctors often complain about the lack of time for satisfactory consultations in which all participants adequately understand the information. This can frustrate patients' expectations since it can provoke unnecessary anxiety through lack of understanding, or even misunderstanding, and prevent the patient from making informed decisions. In addition, when patients are in emotional shock, they are not in a good position to understand all the information provided orally in the face-to-face consultation (García-Izquierdo & Muñoz-Miquel 2015). Patients may be given leaflets to take home and read for themselves or discuss with relatives. Links to official bodies or associations webpages, patient blogs, home health manuals, online audio-visual tutorials and popular articles may also provide relevant information and reassurance.

3.2.2 The informed consent and the consultation

Listening to patients and respecting their autonomy is emphasised in all ethical guidance. During the consultation, the interaction between doctor and patient may involve aspects, such as a routine physical examination, that require the patient's consent (see Chapter 2 for more detailed information about this genre). In those cases, consent need not be in writing. As long as patients understand what is proposed, a verbal indication of acceptance can be sufficient (British Medical Association Ethics Department 2013). However, written authorisation is advisable for higher-risk or innovative treatments and is legally required for some procedures, depending on national legislations.

Patients can be faced with more than one medical alternative in risk situations, such as a surgical intervention or a chemotherapy treatment. In order for them to make adequate choices, patients need information to understand what is proposed and why. Standard information provided in written texts in the mother tongue of the patients can be a first step in informing them. Patients may read that information at home, provided it is conveyed in a comprehensible way, and return to the consultation with questions about relevant issues they have not grasped sufficiently. A standard presentation of options, no matter how accurate and evidence based it is, is not very helpful as a final solution. A more personalised approach of what may be effective or appropriate for their particular situation makes more sense to them. That is why patients often need to discuss orally the pros and cons of the different alternatives with their doctors to reach a shared decision and give consent in a fully informed way.

3.2.3 The telephone consultation

In the wake of the pandemic, there was a significant increase in the use of remote consultations through email, videoconferencing and telephone. These modes have some advantages: they enable remote communication when face-to-face medical encounters are not possible, they reduce costs and most people have easy access to telephones and computers. These important advantages, however, come at a price.

In the case of telephone consultations, lack of visual information and physical contact have a negative impact on a number of communicative issues, including diminished trust derived from the difficulty to identify the interlocutors. Checking who the patient is and making sure that the patient knows who the doctor is are necessary initial steps in any encounter. In face-to-face spoken interactions, lip reading plays an important role. Lack of visual input makes understanding oral language a more difficult enterprise.

In addition to that, the impossibility of perceiving and interpreting facial expressions has a negative impact on turn taking and pausing. Empathetic pausing is particularly challenging because the listener does not know whether the doctor is still there in longer pauses. Pace is also affected: the speed at which patients understand spoken information in telephone consultations is affected by the lack of visual input.

Another important challenge is referring to parts of the body. What can easily be sorted out as "It hurts here or there" in face-to-face interactions requires accurate names or explanations which may not be at hand for the patient at the moment of remote communication. Signposting is another challenging area of remote oral interaction. The layout on the page does the sorting out for you of the structure, categories, levels and so on. In face-to-face interactions, signposting can be reinforced through body language. However, over the phone, the tone of voice, pausing in the right places, pace, articulation of vowels and consonants and stress on critical words can signpost and contribute to understanding speech without visual cues.

The fact that both doctors and patients may use jargon or informal language (see Chapter 5), characterised by the use of metaphors, euphemisms, abbreviations, local references or idioms, may also hinder communication. Whenever you say anything, there is the content and there is also a relationship aspect, which affects how you say it, and they both matter because when you are talking to somebody you are building a relationship, good or bad. The closer doctors can align their vocabulary, syntax and prosody to match their patients, the greater the empathy and the more comfortable the interaction for both parties (see Chapter 6).

The absence of linguistic alignment can hinder adequate diagnosis and treatment and increase risks for the patient. Medical interpreters can be useful for reducing language barriers in health care. In a crisis scenario such as the Covid-19 pandemic lockdowns, telephone interpreting emerged when face-to-face or online consultations were not an option. One of the distinctive features of telephone interpreting is its lack of visual information and the sort of oral strategies that come into play to compensate for that visual void in the interaction, such as prosody (intonation, articulation, speed, pauses, pitch) or even voice quality (timbre). The technical equipment and restrictions involved in telephone interpreting affect the way interpreters deal with these remote consultations.

In addition to translating, interpreters need to coordinate the medical encounter. This coordination involves managing the beginning and end as well as turn taking and interrupting the speakers as and when needed in the course of the consultation. Unlike in face-to-face consultation, in mediated telephone consultations, turn taking becomes harder, even harder than in non-mediated consultations. Cutting in to be able to translate can be difficult, and pre-arranging and agreeing on a procedure so that no offence is caused can be necessary so that interpreters can translate. These changes also affect video consultations and are inevitably transforming the way doctors and patients interact and also how medical interpreters and translators work in these remote settings, since they cannot benefit from the cues that non-verbal language provides in face-to-face interactions (Muñoz-Miquel 2019).

3.2.4 Good multimodal practice in the consultation

In patient-centred communication and translation, the interplay and coherence between spoken and written communication can and should be reinforced (Montalt & García-Izquierdo 2016). Generally speaking, good practice guidelines for medical professionals have not been developed across Europe or in the United States or China. In these cases, there is no tradition of guides to good practice common to the entire public health system but rather specific models or recommendations in specific areas (medicines, patient booklets, specific specialities) promoted by various agents, such as hospitals or patient associations. In other countries, however, we find more comprehensive approaches, such as in the United Kingdom, where the National Health Service uses the good practice guidelines framed in the Calgary–Cambridge Guide.

The Calgary–Cambridge Guide was developed by Silverman et al. (1997). It has become an established standard text in communication skills teaching, the first entirely evidence-based textbooks on medical interviewing. Calgary-Cambridge Guide-oriented textbooks explore in detail the specific skills of patient–doctor communication and provide comprehensive evidence of how those skills can improve health outcomes and everyday clinical practice. The Calgary–Cambridge Guide itself is essential reading for learners at all levels (whether medical students, residents or established practitioners) and for facilitators and programme directors. In the framework of this guide, patients are not passive recipients of information. They are active agents in the communication process. This guide clearly highlights the need to combine written information with oral information to improve patient understanding. It is structured as follows:

1) Initiating the session (introduction; obtain personal data; reasons for the consultation; agenda setting).
2) Gathering information (encourage patients to tell their stories, ask questions and leave patient time to answer; observe body language and affect; clarify vague statements; periodically summarise; avoid jargon; encourage patients to express their feelings).
3) Providing structure (summarise a specific line of inquiry to confirm understanding; progress from one section to another using transitional statements).
4) Building the relationship (demonstrate appropriate non-verbal behaviour; accept the legitimacy of patients' views; communicate empathetically; provide support; deal sensitively with embarrassing and disturbing topics; ask permission during physical examinations).
5) Explanation and planning.
6) Closing the session (contract with patient; check that patient agrees and is comfortable with plan).

These sections are further developed into specific tasks, skills and stages. As we can see, the first four stages concentrate on specific aspects of the consultation, which necessarily involve contact between doctor and patient and therefore oral interaction. However, section five, *Explanation and planning*, is particularly relevant to written communication. This section is divided into four major blocks (*Providing the correct amount and type of information; Aiding accurate recall and understanding; Achieving a shared understanding: incorporating the patient's perspective*; and *Planning: shared decision making*).

The guide contains a further section called *Options in explanation and planning*. Point 41 explicitly mentions the advisability of using written communication in the form of texts, diagrams and other visual elements. The need therefore arises for the patient and the doctor to have access to suitable visual and written resources. It is precisely in this recommendation that we find the interplay between oral and written communication. Both translators and interpreters working in or around the consultation need to be aware of these intermodal connections.

Since the patient is a unique individual with a unique experience of illness and health, most of the steps involved in the initial phases of the consultation are inherently oral. Methods such as role playing can help to train future professionals in communication skills that are essential for medical practice. Not only doctors or medical students but also patients, translators and interpreters can benefit from this method to understand how a consultation works.

3.2.5 Fostering communication skills through roleplays

In addition to theoretical and practical knowledge as well as normative frameworks of good practices, both health professionals and students find role playing an adequate tool for learning and improving communication skills with peers and with patients. Role playing refers to acting and speaking as though you are a character in a given situation; a roleplay is the act of dramatising a given communicative situation through dialogue and interaction with other characters (see subsection 7.1.9 in Chapter 7). The focus of role playing is on specific interpersonal interactions and the rational and emotional motivations leading to behaviours, attitudes and decisions of their participants.

The overall aim of role playing is educational, and education in the field of communication is often based on simulation. The purpose of simulation is to offer opportunities to practice the relevant skills, to apply the relevant knowledge and to reflect on the relevant attitudes and values (Skelton 2008). It is used in many disciplines and professions – such as law, business, and telephone interpreting – as a tool to facilitate the acquisition of social and communicative skills. The situations and issues explored in roleplays are open in nature and give rise to several possible interpretations and solutions depending on the individuals and the context involved. Clinical role playing has been shown to promote reflection and insight not only for students in the patient and professional roles but also for peers observing the group sessions. It is a practice that allows participants to explore problems and try out solutions in safe environments that do not deal with real patients. Clinical roleplays facilitate equality and increase students' involvement, self efficacy, and empathic abilities (Rønning & Bjørkly 2019).

For further information on clinical role playing, you can visit one of the leading institutions in the field, the Interactive Studies Unit at the University of Birmingham with its multidisciplinary team with backgrounds in medicine, nursing, education, linguistics, drama, literature and ethics.

TASK 3.1 EXPLORING THE INTERPLAY BETWEEN ORAL AND WRITTEN IN THE CONSULTATION

Materials

You will need the collaboration of a volunteer preferably with no medical background.

You will also need an informed consent form in your language. It can be about any health issue of your choice.

Procedure

1) Ask your volunteer to imagine he or she is a patient in a face-to-face consultation having to make a decision about an important health issue.
2) Ask your volunteer to read the informed consent form and to identify any obscure language in the text, no matter how apparently inconsequential it may seem. It can be a single word, a technical term, a full sentence or paragraph or even a concept or idea that spreads across several sentences or paragraphs. It can also be information that is missing in the text.
3) Encourage the volunteer to ask you questions about any obscure words, sentences, concepts or ideas. Ask the volunteer to be as picky, demanding and challenging as possible.
4) At a later stage, make two lists, one containing the language problems you can fix (such as sentence length or unclear specialised terminology), and the other one containing the specialised knowledge that you would need to discuss with a subject matter expert.
5) Introduce in the texts the improvements that are needed such as avoiding or explaining technical terms, expanding background knowledge, changing the order of paragraphs or adding verbal or visual information.
6) Share the improved version with your volunteer and get feedback from your volunteer. Is this easier? Why? Which solutions work better now? Are there any words you don't like? How could it be improved further?

As we have discussed so far, the interplay between oral and written – as well as between verbal and non-verbal – communication is a crucial element in the consultation, the core patient–doctor genre from which other genres stem. When face-to-face consultations are not practicable, new intermodal challenges arise that need to be properly addressed by writers, translators and interpreters. These challenges become even more pressing with patients with disabilities.

3.3 Accessibility and inclusivity

Many patients experience sensory impairments affecting vision or hearing. These impairments can be inherited or appear later in life as the consequence of a variety of factors, including aging, working conditions and multiple diseases. Other patients may experience difficulties in making sense of verbal language, and written language in particular, not because of sensory impairments but owing to neurological or mental disorders such as Asperger's syndrome or dementia.

For example, there is evidence that many patients with schizophrenia show severe deficits in reading ability (Revheim et al. 2014). As a result, these people can experience marginalisation and exclusion of all sorts, including access to adequate health care. Improving communication addressed to or involving these patients can improve their lives in a number of ways, whereas failure to communicate in appropriate formats can lead to problems with prevention, diagnosis, adherence to treatment and self-monitoring.

Accessible multimodal translation responds to the variability in different recipients' sensory and cognitive capacities to access information and participate in communication. It includes three main areas:

- Audio description, Braille and large print for blind and partially sighted patients.
- Subtitling and interpreting in sign language for deaf and hard-of-hearing patients.
- More recently, intralingual translation to produce user-friendly materials for those with learning difficulties (cognitive diversity).

3.3.1 Blind and partially sighted patients

The WHO estimates that globally, at least 2.2 billion people have a vision impairment or blindness, which means that they find it difficult to access relevant information of all sorts, in particular, about medicine and health care. There are multiple causes, from uncorrected refractive errors and cataracts and age-related macular degeneration to glaucoma, diabetic retinopathy, corneal opacity and trachoma, and one of the consequences, as far as health care and communication are concerned, is barriers to access to relevant information about those and other conditions.

Information about other age-related health issues may also need to be addressed.

In cases of patients with some vision who struggle to read regular print, large or giant print may be a solution. Large print is generally 16- to 18-point in size, whereas giant print is anything larger than that. Owing to their relevance in treatment, documents such as patient information leaflets are likely to be needed in large print.

Another way of overcoming barriers that blind patients encounter is Braille, a system of writing and reading that uses raised dot patterns to represent characters that can be read by touching with the fingertips. Although it is not a language but a code in which many languages – such as Arabic, Chinese, English, Spanish – can be written, it is the primary literacy medium for people who are blind or have severe low vision. The use of Braille is regulated in some health care systems, where pharmaceutical companies must legally respond to requests for alternative formats from patients and their health care professionals.

The inclusion of Braille on pharmaceutical packaging in Europe and the United States is now the norm. European Union Directive 2001/83/EC requires that all products authorised after 30 October 2005 carry Braille identification. Information on pharmaceutical Braille can be very useful for writers and translators. However, visually impaired patients vary a great deal. Some are born blind or lose their sight early in life, whereas others suffer sight loss in old age. Some patients are educated as blind and are introduced to Braille at an early age, and some chose never to learn Braille or, having tried, have never mastered it.

Another of the solutions to overcome these barriers is audio description, spoken narration that is added to make visual content accessible. These descriptions can be offered live or can be made available in recorded form as part of an audio guide. Audio description began in the cultural and entertainment sectors: in performing arts such as opera or theatre, it describes body language and movements of actors and singers as well as props and lighting effects; in film or television, it describes the visual aspects of the action and place. Through an additional soundtrack, the visual images that carry meaning or value for the sighted viewer are audibly conveyed to those without sight.

Audio description is also used in a variety of other contexts such as museums, architectural and archaeological sites, art galleries and live performances. The guidelines presented by audio description projects ADLAB and ADLAB PRO (Rémael et al. 2015) are meant to offer reliable, consistent, research-based guidelines for making arts and media products accessible to the blind and visually impaired. In addition, the World Wide Web Consortium helps people understand and create audio description of visual information for new and existing videos in the world wide web. Patients can benefit from many of these developments. Thus, health authorities and communicators should consider them when making multimodal choices to address blind and partially sighted patients in an inclusive way.

3.3.2 Deaf and hard of hearing patients

The WHO estimates that 466 million people worldwide suffer disabling hearing loss and that this figure will increase to 900 million people by 2050. Hearing loss may result from genetic factors, complications at birth such as birth asphyxia, certain infectious diseases, chronic ear infections, the inappropriate use of particular drugs during pregnancy, exposure to excessive noise and ageing. Deafness and hearing loss often put people at a disadvantage. As happens with other sensory and cognitive minorities, if this disadvantage is not properly addressed and catered to, discrimination can marginalise the deaf and hard of hearing from many social spheres and public life.

Captioning and subtitling for the deaf and hard-of-hearing has its origins in television, with the pioneering work of the BBC, which introduced its Ceefax teletext service in 1972. Since the 1970s, reception studies of film, television and other audiovisual products and services have paid particular attention to subtitling. One of the original concerns was to compare and evaluate the different ways – mainly sign translation and captioning formats – in which information could be conveyed to and understood by deaf people. Over the decades, some researchers focused on determining the optimal speed and other parameters for deaf people to adequately understand captioning. Others looked at correlations between subtitles and speech speed depending on the type of programme, news, soap operas, documentaries, etc. For example, slow subtitles may be appropriate for active location shots and faster subtitles for "studio presentations with a static newsreader" (de Linde & Kay 1999: 76, cited in Romero-Fresco 2016: 207–208).

More recently, eye tracking has been used to analyse the eye movements of deaf viewers with different degrees of hearing loss in terms of time spent on subtitles and images, time spent lip-reading speakers and genre of audiovisual product. Issues such as preference for block subtitles over scrolling subtitles, linguistic complexity of subtitles, actual comprehension by viewers, the need for international harmonisation, the diversity of hearing-impaired communities around the world and the quality of live subtitles are also current issues in access to communication for deaf and hard of hearing people (Romero-Fresco 2016).

The pioneering work on the effectiveness of subtitles, both in media and film studies and later in audiovisual translation, cannot be overlooked in the field of health care communication, writing and translation. Deaf and hard of hearing patients interacting in clinical settings can benefit from many of the advances in audiovisual translation. However, the specific complexities of clinical communication that make it different from the entertainment industry of film and television need to be critically considered.

3.3.3 Patients with learning difficulties

Patients with learning difficulties may have unique communication needs that require special attention and adaptation by health care professionals, translators, writers and interpreters. Addressing these needs is critical to ensuring that individuals with learning difficulties receive equitable and accessible health care.

Some considerations for the communication needs of patients with learning difficulties include using clear, simple, straightforward language; avoiding medical terminology and jargon; using visual aids, such as pictures or diagrams, to supplement verbal explanations; repeating important information multiple times and reinforcing key points and providing information in accessible formats, such as large print and audio or video formats to accommodate diverse learning styles. In face-to-face communication, it may be useful to use interactive and engaging techniques such as role playing or demonstrations, and to check understanding periodically.

TASK 3.2 CHALLENGES FOR VISUALLY IMPAIRED PATIENTS AND CONSEQUENCES FOR WRITERS AND TRANSLATORS

Procedure and materials

1) Watch this video www.rnib.org.uk/eye-health/your-guide-diabetes-related-eye-conditions/managing-diabetes-sight-loss and identify the information that the patient, who has diabetic retinopathy (an eye condition that can cause vision loss and blindness), needs and the strategies she uses to obtain it.
2) Read the article "Usability of Medical Devices for Patients With Diabetes Who Are Visually Impaired or Blind" (Heinemann et al. 2016) and consider the following questions:

   - Why is there a need for a legal requirement for manufacturers to provide accessible/user-friendly technical aids for visually impaired and blind patients with diabetes?
   - What advantages do these aids bring both for patients and the health system?

- Normally we assume that the text we produce will be read by a reader. Now imagine you are writing or translating a text addressed to someone who can hear but cannot see and that your text will be read aloud and recorded for your hearers. Considering that you cannot rely on layout and illustrations, would you write in a different way? If so, what would the differences be?
- How do you think your writing or translation can influence the way the text will be read aloud in the target language of your hearers and help them to understand the information?

In the field of patient-centred translation and communication, we can borrow relevant knowledge and experience from other areas such as audio-visual translation. As has been pointed out, subtitling is a rich professional and research field that offers technical solutions that can be adapted to health communication. Dubbing is another field from which to learn and benefit. Translators of scripts of films and other audio-visual products face the challenge of having to write in a register and style which will be read aloud by actors and heard by the target hearers/viewers. Their experience and concepts can surely be relevant for writers and translators involved in audio description in the health sector.

3.4 Expanding modes and formats

Accessible, user-friendly voice-based technologies are not limited to the visually impaired but can also be of great help to any patient. For example, this is what Olivia, a patient with diabetes, says about the communication problems she faces:

> A diagnosis with diabetes is a lot. It's easy to forget all the information that is thrown at you by your doctor or get lost in the endless pamphlets of facts that you come home with. You may be asking yourself: What should I eat? What are the symptoms of high blood sugar? Should I exercise after I eat?

This reflects some of the common information worries expressed by patients. Big pharmaceutical companies such as Roche have developed new voice technologies to address these needs, as for example, Sulli the Diabetes Guru. This is a free, on-demand voice assistant available through Amazon Alexa and Google Assistant for people newly diagnosed with type 2 diabetes. Solutions such as Sulli incorporate knowledge about specific diseases into accessible user-friendly voice experiences. They answer questions, offer lifestyle advice and enable users to set reminders to take medication or locate the nearest blood glucose monitor retailer.

3.4.1 Digitalisation and eHealth

The unprecedented spread of digital technology as well as its increased capabilities are making a huge impact in many different fields including health care. New ways of providing access to digital health resources are emerging, and the crisis driven by Covid-19 accelerated this transformation. A pandemic requires global information and communication strategies, in particular those dealing with prevention and response. The internet allows access to sources of information that can influence behaviour and habits, which has the potential to transform medicine and patient care in a broad sense.

As seen in Chapter 2 (see subsection 2.4.1), eHealth is made up of tools and services that use information and communication technologies to improve such things as prevention, diagnosis and treatment and to monitor and manage lifestyle habits that impact health. Telemedicine, mobile health, artificial intelligence-enabled medical devices and virtual reality tools are examples of changes which are reshaping how patients and consumers interact with health professionals, how their data are shared among providers and how decisions are made about treatment plans and health outcomes.

Electronic health resource access is closely linked to the notion of the *digital patient*, who is proactive, empowered, informed, connected and critical (see Chapter 4). Digital patients focus on prevention and maintenance and often demand information about their health. Digitalisation and the digital patient can enhance the possibilities of personalised medicine, which involves tailoring the medical treatment to the individual characteristics of each patient or group of patients.

Personalised medicine's basic statement is that everyone is unique, which requires a move away from a one-size-fits-all approach to one that adopts a treatment strategy based on the unique genetic profile of each patient. Digital technologies can be used to collect the large amounts of data that are needed to support personalized medicine. They can also be used to analyse the data that is collected and identify patterns that might be relevant to personalised medicine.

For example, algorithms can be used to identify genetic variations that are associated with certain diseases or to predict how a patient is likely to respond to a particular treatment. Digital technologies can also be used to deliver personalised medicine interventions, including personalised medication recommendations or lifestyle changes that might be beneficial for their health. Finally, according to the European Commission's 2018 Communication on Digital Health and Care, digital technologies can empower citizens, making it easier for them to play a greater role in the management of their own health.

While much is positive about eHealth, challenges remain. Not everyone has access to the technology or the skills to use it. Even more broadly, more than half of the world's population does not have access to basic health care, and according to the WHO, around 100 million people are pushed into extreme poverty because they have to pay for health care. That is why all United Nations member states have agreed to work towards achieving universal health coverage by 2030 as part of the Sustainable Development Goals. Universal health coverage aims to ensure that everyone has access to the health services they need, when and where they need them without financial hardship. It covers the full range of essential health services, from health promotion to prevention, treatment, rehabilitation and palliative care.

In recent years, eHealth has also been developed in response to the growing need for universal health coverage. More than half of WHO Member States have an eHealth strategy, and 90% of eHealth strategies refer to the goals of universal health coverage or its key elements (WHO 2016). This means that digital infrastructures are increasingly available for use in humanitarian crises (Montalt 2021).

3.4.2 New multimodal genres arising from digitalisation

Technology has facilitated combining different formats and media: audio, video, graphics, texts, web sites, voice-recognition devices, apps, leaflets, animation pictures, chats. They fulfil different needs: broadening patients' and health providers' access to relevant health information, enhancing the quality of care, reducing health care errors, increasing collaboration and encouraging the adoption of healthy behaviour. This means that many written documents that already exist have had to be adapted to fit into the requirements of this new multimodal environment of the digital age. In addition to apps (see subsection 2.4.1 in Chapter 2), some examples are electronic informed consent, electronic health records and electronic prescriptions.

The information in electronic consent documents is the same as on written forms but may be expanded to include images, audio, video, diagrams, reports, callout boxes, narration, a digital signature and so forth. These additional features are meant to help patients to understand the text and empower them to make better informed decisions. The electronic health record is a digital version of a patient's medical history and includes among other things diagnoses, treatment plans, test results and immunisation dates. It is made available instantly and confidentially to health professionals and can improve patient care as they enhance the accuracy and clarity of the records and reduce the incidence of error. Electronic prescribing is aimed at optimising and eliminating possible human error from the prescribing process. It also facilitates the collection of data for national health services, which it is hoped will lead to more effective and efficient long-term planning and policies better suited to people's needs.

Owing to the Covid-19 pandemic, many people started to avoid hospitals, and telemedicine became the new normal. Increasingly commercial enterprises are developing remote monitoring and telemedicine. Societal change in conjunction with new technologies are reshaping the clinical consultation as we know it. As seen in subsection 3.2.3, face-to-face consultations are rapidly giving way to telephone and video consultations, and online texting in chats between doctors and patients. Interactive portals allow patients to book appointments online and receive reminders and chatbots address frequently asked questions for patients.

Wearables are another important innovation: smart health watches; fitness trackers, which monitor heart rate, calorie expenditure, mileage and sleep quality; skin patches, which provide information such as the user's blood pH, sweat rate or blood sugar level; hearables, which can measure heart rate, speed, distance and body temperature; oximeters, which are used by patients with respiratory illnesses and wearable ECG monitors, which measure an electrocardiogram and send the reading to the user's doctor. These are some of the options which enable patients to monitor their own health and participate more actively in their own care. Wearable technologies can foster patient-centred care by placing knowledge and control back in the hands of the patient: they measure and track their own health metrics and are empowered to bring this information to their doctors to help guide treatment plans and therefore play a more active role in their own health care.

While the appearance of so many different types of communication devices is to be welcomed, it is also important to consider to what extent they are in fact useful and user friendly. Producers, designers and indeed translators need to ask themselves questions such as whether they can be accessed by all intended users or whether they provide information which is relevant and easy to understand.

TASK 3.3 EXPLORING HEALTH APPS

Procedure and materials

1) Go to https://smokefreeapp.com/ and download the app. The Smoke Free app (<https://smokefreeapp.com/>) is designed to help smokers give up their habit. It was developed using behaviour change techniques which

had been found effective in face-to-face behavioural support programmes and provides users with helpful strategies.

2) Have the designers written in plain English? Can you find examples of user-centred language in it?
3) What types of actions are users asked to perform?
4) Consider: (i) Which communication strategies (e.g. ways of addressing the reader; see Chapter 4) do you think are effective for achieving the purpose? Why? (ii) Which of the strategies do you think could be improved? How?
5) Now, choose some of the most relevant information for the user and translate it into your target language trying to make sure that your translation is usable.

In this chapter, we have discussed multimodality in terms of interaction, accessibility and technology. We have provided a selected sample of multimodal resources at the service of patients' needs and their involvement in health care. Representation and communication are largely rooted in verbal language but go beyond it. The meaning-making resources used by patients in different personal and contextual circumstances are diverse. All of these resources are socially, culturally and technologically shaped, which means that the inventory of multimodal resources in different cultures and societies is variable and dynamic; that is, technological innovation gives rise to new ones that gradually come to the fore, and old ones are either transformed or disappear.

Many of these resources are produced in specific contexts, such as a country, a health system or a health organisation. Others are designed for a globalised world, where authors and translators need to consider not only users but also the possibilities and limitations of the technology available in particular contexts and situations. Similarly, developers of the new multimodal resources are designing and developing their innovations in the knowledge that they will need to be translated into many different languages. Controlled and simplified language is therefore a necessary prerequisite for making all these devices translatable into any language. In addition, machine translation and post-editing are increasingly used to make all resources and devices available to patients in any language. The extent to which these highly standardised languages clash with more personalised, subjective, culturally bound, patient-centred care communication and translation remains to be seen.

It is debatable to what extent all technological innovations really empower patients. In some cases, they probably do, but in others, efficiency, speed and customer satisfaction are the driving forces. There is also a worrying ethical dimension to these technologies. Digital devices that transmit personal data easily and at the touch of a button come at a high price: the data are transmitted to a legitimate health authority but also stored and controlled by the technology companies. Personal medical data can then be used by insurance companies in ways that are not in the patient's best interests. A more patient-centred, humanised approach to communication should ensure patient privacy and confidentiality at every point in the communication continuum.

Further reading

Ainsworth, S.; Griffiths, D.; Macrory, G.; Pahl, K. *Multimodality and Multilingualism: Towards an Integrative Approach*; Multilingual Matters, 2023.

Borg, K.; Boulet, M.; Smith, L.; Bragge, P. Digital Inclusion & Health Communication: A Rapid Review of Literature. *Health Communication*, 2019, *34* (11), 1320–1328.

Butcher, C. J.; Hussain, W. Digital Healthcare: The Future. *Future Healthcare Journal*, 2022, *9* (2), 113–117.

Lyles, C. R.; Fruchterman, J.; Youdelman, M.; Schillinger, D. Legal, Practical, and Ethical Considerations for Making Online Patient Portals Accessible for All. *American Journal of Public Health*, 2017, *107* (10), 1608–1611.

Neighbour, R. *The Inner Consultation: How to Develop an Effective and Intuitive Consulting Style*; CRC Press, 2018

Neves, J. Translation and Accessibility: The Translation of Everyday Things. In *The Routledge Handbook of Translation and Methodology*; Zanettin, F.; Rundle, C., Eds.; Routledge, 2022; pp. 441–456.

Meng, J.; Bouillon, P.; Seligman, M. *Translation Technology in Accessible Health Communication*; Cambridge University Press: Cambridge, 2023.

4

ANALYSING YOUR TARGET AUDIENCE

Overview of chapter

The centrality of the patient in the famous quote by William Osler at the beginning of the Introduction of this book is also relevant to communicators, pointing to a shift in focus from biomedical knowledge to multiple audiences and how they shape and use that knowledge in different ways in real communication. This chapter addresses one of the most vital factors when making decisions in patient-centred translation and communication: the target audience and how we address it.

When translating or writing for patients it is often overlooked that texts will not be perceived in the same way by readers of different ages, levels of health literacy or cultural backgrounds, to mention just a few of the factors that may affect how audiences respond to the information they receive. Although in translation studies *skopos* (Nord 1997) theory has provided a set of concepts that have shifted the centre of attention from the source text/author to the target text/reader, some further refinement of *skopos* is needed in the context of patient-centred communication. The notions of user-centred translation (Suojanen et al. 2015) and audience design (Bell 1984; Mason 2000) underlie the entire chapter as well as the claim that there is not a general category of patient but rather, many subgroups with specific needs that should be considered. In this regard, a parallel between translating/writing for patients and personalised medicine can be drawn. The difficulty of singularising and tailoring texts to all patient's expectations and needs must be acknowledged.

Addressing someone involves the act of communicating or interacting with them, and the way you do it can vary depending on the mode of

DOI: 10.4324/9780429299698-5

communication (oral, written, multimodal), the social and cultural context where it takes place – in which codes of politeness play a role – and the specific communicative situation or genre (Section 4.1). To characterise the communicative situations, several variables are presented: participants, relations among participants, channel, processing circumstances, setting and communicative purpose (Section 4.2). In order to make adequate choices in your text, when analysing your audience (Section 4.3), you can zoom in and focus on several coexisting roles: recipient, addressee, reader, user, patient and beneficiary. One crucial issue when analysing your audience is understanding the variety of patients' profiles and their particular needs (Section 4.4). Finally, some recommendations are provided to address your audiences in a patient-centred way (Section 4.5).

4.1 Audiences and genres addressed to patients

Throughout her life as a patient with diabetes, Olivia has been addressed many times by health professionals for a variety of reasons, from asking questions about her health to providing therapeutic advice to getting permission for a procedure. Normally she is addressed in her mother tongue, except when she has been abroad and an interpreter has not been available. In these situations, she has struggled because of the difficulties of not fully understanding the health professionals she is talking to or not being fully understood. The degree of formality with which Olivia is addressed varies depending on the situation. For example, she may be addressed less formally or even colloquially in a face-to-face conversation with the doctor, where she likes to be called personally by her name, whereas she may be addressed more formally on an informed consent form, where she is referred to in a more depersonalised way as a standard patient.

Being addressed and addressing others – both as individual or collective audiences – is a fundamental aspect of communication and society. From our first breath in life, we are addressed by our parents and gradually learn to respond to them in our early development; later, we learn to respond to other members of our family and friends, teachers at school and colleagues at work. We are constantly being addressed in face-to-face or remote interactions through printed or online texts; and because we are culturally aware of what it means to be addressed privately or publicly, we are able to understand and make sense of messages from our positions in this situated process of address in addition to our individual cognitive abilities.

4.1.1 The active role of the audience

Traditionally, rhetoric has treated the audience as passive (see Section 1.1 in Chapter 1) and the writer or speaker as active, as if communication were a linear and unidirectional process and the audience were radically detached from the previous stages of this process. Today, in medical and health care communication, the audience is still predominantly seen as passive. In the case of patients as recipients of medical care, this is crystal clear: they are seen only as passive recipients and health professionals as active providers. However, this passivity, although deeply rooted in many health care systems and cultures, does not benefit patients in terms of communication and care.

Bakhtin (1986) offers an alternative, active view of communicative roles that can be useful for a critical understanding of audiences in which genres can be seen as utterances, that is, acts of communication addressed to specific audiences. He argues that words have an internal dialogism in which they are directed towards an answer and are influenced by the answering words they anticipate. Accordingly, when analysing audiences, we should focus on utterances (units of expression tied to specific acts of speaking or writing in given communicative situations) rather than sentences (grammatical units with specific formal structures) because audiences are intrinsically implied in utterances, whereas sentences are merely acontextual linguistic structures. Even when we make terminological choices based on who is going to read them – in our case, patients – we are actually thinking of medical terms as utterances directed to a specific target reader, and in our choices, we are anticipating their responses.

Utterances not only contain information but also reflect attitudes and establish relationships. Utterances are characterised by the fact that they are always directed to someone, that is, by their *addressivity*; at the same time, they are always received by someone, that is, they characterised by their *receptivity*. Audiences are regulated by responsive, active understanding of all kinds of situations (see Chapter 2). For these reasons, in this chapter, we are interested in both oral and written utterances rather than sentences.

Suggestions for task. Addressing patients in different situations

How are patients addressed in different situations (a medical consultation, a patient information leaflet, a health campaign, an informed consent form, an advert of a medicine, a patient's association website, etc.) in your health culture? Discuss the degree of formality, the attitudes, and the types of relationships that the different modes of address entail. Compare them with other languages and health cultures.

4.1.2 Audiences and genres

The act of addressing shapes the style and the register (and with it the terminological choices we make) of genres, as well as the role of the addressee. However, this does not necessarily mean that it is done in the best possible way for the addressee, in our case, in a patient-centred way. Many institutionalised genres, such as some of those described in Chapter 2, place the addressee in a position that is often not optimal for the patient, that is, not patient centred. Addressers, who are not necessarily competent communicators, often position themselves in a role of power and dominance over patients, with direct consequences for language and communication.

As well as being governed by formal conventions that determine how we write or translate within them, genres also reflect contextual and situational features such as the profile and role of the participants. Consider Olivia in the doctor's consultation: even before she enters it, both the doctor and Olivia have pre-established roles, and both have expectations for how they should behave and interact within those roles. In fact, both behave and interact according to implicit and explicit norms or cultural scripts that are taken for granted in such a situation.

These norms of communication can be clearly seen, for example, in the way the medical history is taken. In medical schools, students are taught what to ask, in what order, with what questions and so on (e.g. the questions contained in the Calgary-Cambridge Guide; see subsection 3.1.1 in Chapter 3). Medical students learn about the consultation as an act of communication or genre both formally through university textbooks and experientially as residents, observing experienced doctors at work. In addition to these pre-established communication norms, the individual personality of each health professional plays a crucial role in the way they address patients.

If the patient and the doctor meet in a different situation outside the consultation – that is, in another genre such as an informal conversation outside the hospital – their expectations and norms will be different, and they will communicate in a different way. Genres regulate communication, both in face-to-face interactions, or remotely through texts, whether it is intralingually or interlingually. In the history and development of each genre, the presence, identity and role of the participants have become entrenched and crystallised in specific forms of addressivity and receptivity. Using a particular genre often means accepting and playing by the rules of that genre.

Taking the informed consent as a case in focus, the following questions point to some relevant issues that communicators should consider: who prepares a consent form in the context of a clinical trial, and from what perspective? For what purpose? And what identities and roles does it create for the promoter, the sponsor and the addressee? For the promoter – a research team, a pharmaceutical laboratory, a health care organisation, etc. – the priority is to *obtain* the consent of the participant so that the legal requirements can be met and the clinical trial can be conducted and completed. The participant's ultimate role is merely to *give* consent. This is what we might call the pragmatic template or script of this particular genre, responding to a medico-legal requirement. The sponsor of the trial is also the sponsor of communication within and around the trial.

Each genre (see Chapter 2) is embedded in a given communicative situation, and writers and translators can benefit from considering how language, in particular style and register in each genre reflect situationality. In principle, each genre is geared towards and responds to the real needs of a specific audience. However, in the genres used in patient-centred communication, this is not always the case. A better understanding of the situation and the audience they are addressing can help communicators make more patient-centred choices.

Suggestions for task. Exploring addressivity in specific genres

Explore the genres in Chapter 2 in your target language and consider how patients are typically addressed and what role they are given within each genre. Discuss how the typical way of addressing the patients in a particular genre could be improved.

4.2 Characterising the situation

Any health professional, patient, writer, translator or interpreter who is in a position to produce texts addressed to patients or to mediate interactions with patients can benefit from considering not only the words themselves but also the communicative situation and its different components and characteristics, as discussed in Chapter 2. A useful framework for analysing such features of the situation would include the following (Biber & Conrad 2019):

- Participants
- Relations among participants
- Channel
- Processing circumstances
- Setting
- Communicative purpose

4.2.1 Participants

In any situation in which we are involved as communicators, there may be several participants, mainly the sender, the receiver and the interlingual and intercultural mediator. In patient-centred translation and communication, senders typically include health professionals, health authorities, researchers, the media and other patients (e.g. patient narratives).

As we argued in Chapter 2, in addition to being the primary audience of the genres we have presented, patients may also be the producers and addressers of the text in the case of patient narratives. In other cases (e.g. the medical consultation), where the patient is the main source of personal information, the roles of addresser and addressee are ideally shared between patient and doctor. In these cases, patients are in control of what information they want to share, with whom and how. In this chapter, we are particularly interested in the participants, more specifically, the audience. In our patient-centred approach, the audience consists primarily of patients but also includes family members, carers and the general public. We will now focus on the recipient as an addressee.

According to audience design theorists, the *addressee* is the intended listener or reader (Bell 1984; Mason 2000). The concept of addressee in patient-centred communication is not always straightforward (see subsection 4.3.1), and further conceptual refinement may be useful. In addition to the addressee, we can consider other related concepts. Consider, for example, a medical consultation in which the patient is accompanied by a relative. Although the doctor is addressing the patient, the relative is known to the doctor and is a ratified participant in the consultation. Bell (1984) and Mason (2000) call this role *auditor*. Depending on the situation and the strategy chosen, the interpreter can be either an auditor or an addressee. Auditors are both known to the speaker and ratified participants but not addressed directly. They should be considered when addressing patients in their presence.

Consider a biopsy report written by a pathologist who gives it to the patient, who in turn gives it to the consultant who requested the test in the first place. In this situation, the patient is known to be present by the pathologist but is neither directly addressed nor a ratified participant. A similar situation occurs with medical reports (see subsection 2.3.5 in Chapter 2), which can often be accessed and read by patients but are not addressed to them. We call this the *overhearer* (known by the speaker to be present but neither directly addressed nor a ratified participant) (Bell 1984; Mason 2000). Finally, when patients read a research paper, the authors are unaware of their presence. This is called an *eavesdropper* (whose presence is not known to the speaker) (Bell 1984; Mason 2000). These concepts may provide relevant clues as to how language can be shaped to best suit its addressees.

Similarly to biopsy reports and medical reports, in other diagnostic genres, such as blood tests or ultrasound reports, the patient is not the addressee of the texts but someone through whose hands they often pass and who can therefore read them but without the ability to interpret them correctly. In general, diagnostic genres require expert knowledge for their correct clinical interpretation. Without such expert knowledge, the patient is unable to infer the meaning of such diagnostic tests and is likely to misinterpret them. The extent to which these texts can be simplified and made available in two different versions – one for doctors and one for patients – is open to discussion.

Suggestions for task. Discussing addressees in diagnostic genres

Discuss with your colleagues or classmates whether diagnostic genres such as those mentioned above (biopsy report, ultrasound report) should be addressed to patients and written accordingly. Why? Why not?

4.2.2 Relationships

Once the participants have been identified, the next step is to describe how they relate and interact with each other. Genres, texts, communication and knowledge only exist in relationships and dialogue, and interactiveness is a key concept. At one extreme, there are situations where all participants are present and can respond directly to each other; this is the case of a medical consultation. At the other extreme are situations where participants do not share the here and now; they are far apart in time or space or both, such as a patient information leaflet. Written texts addressed to patients sometimes reflect a kind of remote interactivity, for example in the form of the questions and answers we often find in patient information leaflets, in which the addresser, a medically authorised participant, anticipates the relevant questions and answers them, such as when to take the medicine, in what quantities or the possible side effects.

Another relevant consideration is the fact that there are asymmetries between patients and health professionals. In institutionalised health care contexts, doctors play a dominant social role based on the authority conferred by their expertise, professional experience and status within the institution. Patients, for their part, tend to assume a passive role, subordinate to the authority of the doctor or nurse. Part of the patient's passivity may stem from fatalism – that is, their view of their own limited self-efficacy – or from complete trust in health professionals. While patients have the knowledge of their personal experiences of illness, the professionals have the biomedical knowledge of the disease, which has a higher social status. These socio-professional asymmetries shape the patient-doctor relationship, directly influence communication and regulate its development (García-Izquierdo & Montalt 2013). Issues such as interpersonal distancing, the degree of terminological complexity or the default national language used in written texts and oral interactions are directly influenced by these asymmetries and need to be taken into account when communicating with patients.

4.2.3 Channels

Specific media directly influence the linguistic forms used by health professionals, patients, writers, translators or interpreters. Writing original texts or translations for a website offers different possibilities (e.g. links to other texts) than writing for a printed document that is physically reproduced, distributed and used. The use of links to other websites or the inclusion of video to complement the verbal message changes the way users navigate and process information. Similarly, writing for an app imposes different constraints and limitations that other channels do not (see Chapter 2). Likewise, when interpreting a patient–doctor interaction over the phone or online, there are a number of issues to consider that are not present or are handled differently in face-to-face interpreting, such as eye contact or turn taking.

4.2.4 Processing circumstances

Processing circumstances involve both sender and addressee and relate to the production and comprehension of the text. In health care, patients are often vulnerable. Circumstances can vary enormously, from a domestic situation in which an individual patient follows instructions to take a medicine prescribed by a doctor to the response to a population-wide pandemic. Processing circumstances often have an emotional dimension (see Chapter 6) that needs to be taken into account. Consider, for instance, reading an informed consent form in the emergency department just before undergoing a complicated surgical procedure or receiving bad news in the consultation. In these examples, the circumstances in which the text is processed or the interaction takes place are crucial. Emotional distress or even shock may affect how patients understand, misunderstand, remember or, indeed, forget the message.

Suggestions for task. Discussing challenging circumstances when processing information

Discuss with your colleagues or classmates in what other circumstances misunderstandings and lack of understanding and recall can occur due to text processing factors.

4.2.5 Setting

Setting refers to the physical context of communication. Hospitals and other health care settings, such as primary care centres, are common places where communication takes place. Hospitals are complex environments where different spaces coexist, such as waiting rooms, emergency departments, operating theatres, chemotherapy wards or bedrooms, to name a few. Home is also a common place for patients to engage in communication and practical tasks related to self-management of their health issues, such as taking medication, following a diet, checking blood pressure or reporting symptoms or other health-related data through telephone consultations, apps or websites. The home is also sometimes the place for palliative and end-of-life care, where communication becomes a critical factor in the emotional well-being of both the patient and the family. Finally, public spaces – both physical and online – are the settings for public health campaigns aimed at society as a whole.

4.2.6 *Communicative purpose*

The communicative purposes of both senders and receivers are truly diverse and lie on a broad continuum. They include taking a medicine safely and effectively; making an informed decision about a procedure; sharing a personal story about health and illness; learning more about a particular disease; providing relevant information to health professionals; understanding the results of a test; changing a health-related habit; adhering to treatment more effectively or making lifestyle changes to improve health, to name but a few.

4.3 Analysing the audience

Whether face-to-face or remote, individual or collective, audiences are complex entities to understand, analyse and engage with effectively. Audience analysis can help us refine our understanding of the participants we are targeting in specific genres and situations and make better decisions about the target text or interaction. Audience analysis involves identifying the audience and tailoring a speech or text to their interests, level of understanding, attitudes and beliefs. An audience-centred approach is important because the effectiveness of communication will be enhanced if the presentation is designed and delivered appropriately. Identifying the audience through extensive research is often difficult precisely because the audience is remote and adapting to it often requires a healthy use of imagination. In this section, we discuss some relevant audience concepts and present a selection of parameters that can be used to identify and analyse the types of patients we are targeting and addressing in real communication.

4.3.1 *Dissecting the idea of the audience and its multiple layers of reception*

When we zoom in on the audience, we can capture its complexity through several overlapping concepts that coexist in the same person of the audience in patient-centred communication: recipient, addressee, reader, user, patient and beneficiary. We argue that these distinctions can be relevant for increasing awareness of the different perspectives that converge on the audience, making better decisions in the process of creating the target text and refining the final result.

Receivers are simply those who receive the message, whether or not they were the intended recipients. Olivia, the imaginary patient we introduced in Chapter 2, has a brother who might read the patient information leaflet of one of the medicines she is taking, but Olivia is the intended recipient of the information, so she is the addressee. Addressing someone in a text means directing the language or making an explicit appeal to that person or group of people. Addressees are therefore embedded and reflected in texts. The tenor, register and style of a text depend largely on the addressee. Writers and translators must ensure that they address their addressees in the most effective and affective way, including the appropriate level of comprehensibility for the patient (see Chapter 5) and the appropriate interpersonal relationship in terms of empathy and alignment with their needs and interests (see Chapter 6).

When recipients read the target text, they become *readers*. Reading refers to the role of actually reading the text and processing the information it contains and is influenced by the level of literacy. In order for Olivia to read the text, she needs to be familiar with the code – that is, the language – and the mode or modes found in the text, verbal, visual, oral, and so on. Reading is not a passive process but one in which readers are constantly responding to the text, or even co-creating meaning. Responsive reading is reflected in a wide range of responses. Olivia could stop reading because the text is not relevant or comprehensible, or she could read it carefully and engage with it because it contains the information she is looking for and is expressed in a way that triggers her active response. Over the years, readers accumulate experience of reading different types of texts or different genres and varieties of language. They therefore have expectations about the register, style and terminology of the text. Readers also have intentions about what to do with the information they read.

The role of the *user* (Suojanen et al. 2015) focuses on what readers do with the information they find in the text, either as they read it or after they have read it. For example, if Olivia is reading a patient information leaflet before taking a medicine that the doctor has prescribed for a persistent cough, she needs clear instructions about the amount of medicine – number of pills, etc. – she should take and how often. Readers are users of information in that they mostly read for practical purposes, such as understanding medical concepts, performing certain actions or achieving health goals. They need to be addressed in a way that enables them to fulfil their purposes and become competent users. From this perspective, as patient-centred communicators, we write words and sentences, and at the same time, we address our audience through utterances that shape the language we use and the structural, stylistic, and terminological choices that we make. Choosing the appropriate flow of information, syntax or word is an act of addressing someone.

As users, patients often read texts and process information in a selective way. Their level of health literacy influences the way they understand and make sense of the information (Berkman et al. 2010). They skip over the parts they consider irrelevant and focus on the sequences that contain the information they are looking for. Depending on their needs and purposes, and the circumstances in which they find themselves, patients have priorities and limitations and process information in different ways. It is very difficult, if not impossible, to anticipate them all, but Figure 4.1 gives a general idea of how they make sense of information and text.

The role of the patient is central to our main argument in this book. Patients are generally recipients, addressees, readers and users who are experiencing illness and are vulnerable. In addition, patients are constantly interacting with health professionals, and these interactions are often asymmetrical, with the patients' role being subordinated, as noted above.

Finally, Olivia benefits from the health care system through her participation in communication. The role of the *beneficiary* is linked to the fiduciary nature

Access

- Patient asks questions.
- Patient skip-searches for information likely to contain the answers.

Interpretation

- Patient understands the verbal and non-verbal information.
- Patient integrates the verbal and non-verbal information.
- Patient infers personal relevance.

Application

- Patient integrates understanding with personal beliefs, values and attitudes.
- Patient determines appropriate decisions and actions.
- Patient devises an action plan with subgoals and necessary steps.
- Patient carries out all steps in plan, monitoring outcomes.
- If monitoring yields a mismatch between subgoals and attainment, the patient formulates a new question and repeats the process.

FIGURE 4.1 Stages in the reading process.

Source: adapted from Wright (1999) and Montalt and González (2007).

of both health care and health communication, where health professionals and communicators are entrusted to act in the patient's best interests (Mehlman 2015; Montalt 2022). Beneficiary thus refers to the fact that patients will benefit from the overall ethical orientation, the behaviour and the specific linguistic and textual choices made by health professionals, translators, writers and interpreters. Communicating with an audience in mind means considering these different roles or levels of reception. It is therefore important to analyse the different dimensions that converge in any act of text-mediated communication and in the production of a written or multimodal text.

4.3.2 Audience expectations

When people become audience members of a text or speech, they bring expectations about the occasion, the topic and the speaker or writer into the act of communication. One of the most basic expectations of any lay audience is to be addressed in their native language. For a writer or speaker, addressing an audience in their mother tongue is a way of recognising them, both individually and collectively, as members of a linguistic and cultural community and thus of acknowledging their identity (García-Izquierdo & Montalt 2022).

Other expectations are based on previous experience in the same situation. For example, in clinical trials, participants are informed before agreeing to take part. Violating the audience's expectations can have a negative impact on the effectiveness of the speech or text. Imagine that a group of participants in a clinical trial are asked to read and sign a consent form. They will expect to be informed about the experiment they are about to take part in, for example, what is being tested or who is sponsoring the experiment and for what purpose and in particular what are possible side effects.

Audience expectations in medical and health care situations are often related to their health and well-being. The credibility and reliability of the author or speaker is an important aspect of the audience's expectations. In health care settings, audiences expect the information they are given to be reliable.

4.3.3 Motivation

Audiences are either voluntary, in which case they are genuinely interested in what a communicator has to say, as in the case of patients; or involuntary, in which case they have no intrinsic interest in the information or the communication process. This may be the case in public health communication, where members of society may be uninterested or even reluctant to receive information. Knowing the difference will help determine how hard a writer or speaker needs to work to engage the audience. Involuntary audiences are notoriously difficult to engage and keep interested in a topic.

Some audiences in medical and health communication are generally most interested in things that directly affect them or their community. An effective writer or speaker must be able to show their audience why the topic they are talking about should be important to them. This is particularly important in health promotion or prevention campaigns.

4.3.4 Focusing on a lay audience

Medical translators and writers often deal with highly specialised genres – such as research articles, clinical guides, summaries of product characteristics or university textbooks – aimed at expert audiences such as researchers, health professionals or health authorities, or at audiences on the way to becoming experts, such as medical students at universities or junior doctors in hospitals. The challenges they face arise from highly specialised content, terminology, information sources or textual conventions. However, for translators and writers interested in health communication, it is crucial to understand the difference between writing for a professional audience and communicating health information to patients and the general public (Figure 4.2).

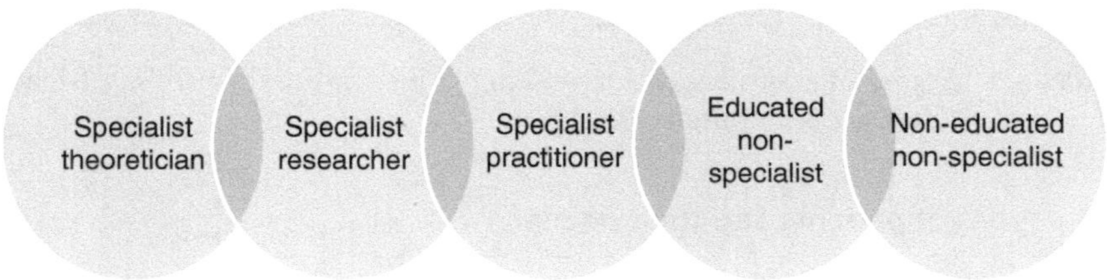

FIGURE 4.2 Continuum of audiences.

As we move to the far right of this continuum and focus on lay audiences with no prior knowledge or experience of medical and health content and communication, the challenges for communicators change and lay friendliness becomes a priority.

Zethsen and Montalt (2022) suggest several micro-strategies for writing or translating (inter- and intralingually) for lay audiences and making a text more lay friendly (see Chapter 5) (Figure 4.3). However, adapting the message to a lay audience is not the same as patronising them by simply telling them what they want to hear or read. Rather, adaptation guides the stylistic and content choices a speaker or writer makes for a presentation or interaction; audience adaptation often involves walking a very fine line between over adaptation and under adaptation.

- Technical terminology. Officialese and technical terminology should generally be avoided and should be translated into lay vocabulary. There are several strategies for determinologising a text and making technical terms easier to understand.
- Syntax. It is often important for a lay reader to know the agent of the sentence. Active voice and verbs instead of nouns usually help the lay reader to understand the medical content better.
- Sentence length. It is generally advisable to break up long sentences up and organise the information they contain in a logical and easy-to-understand way.
- Omission. Information that is not relevant to a lay audience should be omitted, but it goes without saying that the medical expert author of the text to be translated or adapted should be consulted before anything is omitted.
- Explicitation. Lay audiences often lack background knowledge that specialist audiences have or are assumed to have. It is often necessary to make this knowledge explicit in the target text in order to help the reader understand it.
- Structure and graphics. Consider changing the structure of information to create a sequence that is relevant to the target reader. Pictograms and other visual aids may be needed in the target text. Always be aware of cultural differences in the use of images.

FIGURE 4.3 Some microstrategies for making a medical text more lay-friendly (Zethsen & Montalt 2022).

4.4 Types of patients and their needs

Each patient is an individual human being with their own personality and circumstances, and, as we have argued, different roles or levels of reception coexist within them in any act of communication. Whereas health professionals and interpreters deal primarily with individual patients, writers and translators often produce texts for audiences of varying sizes and characteristics. The

TASK 4.1 ANALYSING YOUR AUDIENCES AND CREATING MESSAGES FOR THEM

Procedure and materials

1) Identify and describe different audience segments in the following scenario: a primary care clinic with a diverse patient population seeking information about a common health issue (e.g. diabetes management). Consider factors such as age, cultural background, health literacy, language proficiency and any specific medical conditions relevant to the scenario.

2) Create audience profiles. For each identified audience segment, create detailed audience profiles that include the following information: demographics (age, gender, ethnicity, education level, etc.), health status (existing medical conditions, medication, lifestyle factors, etc.), communication preferences (mother tongue, literacy level, preferred communication channels such as printed text, infographics, video, audio, etc.) and cultural considerations (relevant cultural values and practices).
3) Propose tailored communication strategies for each audience segment based on their profiles. Choose appropriate register considering literacy levels. Select the most effective channels for each audience (e.g. pamphlets, one-to-one consultations, multimedia resources, webpages). Address cultural nuances in communication to ensure relevance and respect.
4) Craft the messages. Develop sample messages or educational materials for each audience segment. Messages should be clear, concise, culturally sensitive and tailored to the specific health issues in the scenario.
5) Discuss your proposal with a colleague or classmate. Get constructive feedback from them and improve the result.
6) Reflect on the whole process.

individual patient takes centre stage in clinical settings, where patient–doctor interaction is the fundamental form of communication. In contrast, public health communication is aimed at a wide range of audiences in society, from specific social groups to society as a whole, as in the case of a pandemic, where ideally every single member of society – whether they are patients or not – is addressed. A broad continuum can thus be established between two extremes: the individual patient and society as a whole (Figure 4.4).

At different points along the continuum, we can find different audiences with different communication needs that pose different types of communication challenges, such as patients of a particular hospital, or a clinical trial, or a patient advocacy group, or suffering from a particular disease, to name but a few. The complexity of audience analysis and targeting lies in the fact that it can vary enormously across a wide range of possibilities, from the individual patient in personalised medicine to the whole of society

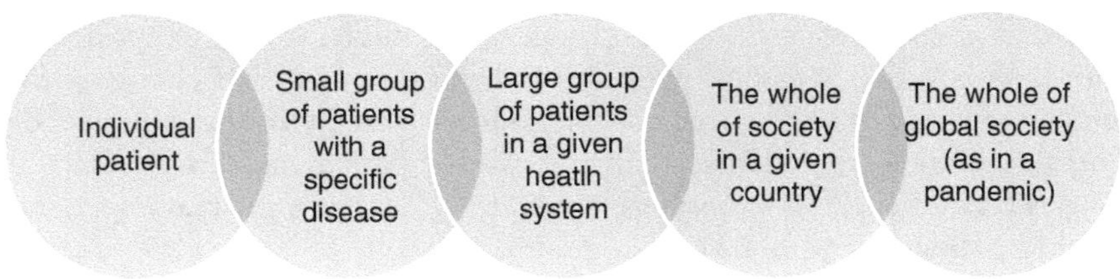

FIGURE 4.4 Continuum of audiences according to size.

in public and global health. The challenges at each point of this continuum are different and require different strategies and solutions. Individualising written information and communication can be difficult because personal circumstances are unique and the role of subjective, cognitive and emotional factors is central.

At the other extreme, addressing society as a whole poses the challenge of not leaving anyone out or behind and finding ways to minimise misunderstanding and ambiguity in messages. Public and global health is a complex arena for multilingual and multicultural communication. Disease outbreaks and emergencies can give rise to crisis situations that require specific actions by affected communities for prevention, containment and control (O'Brien & Federici 2019). Communities need to be informed, motivated and empowered to take the necessary protective actions.

4.4.1 General categories of patient

Patients can be grouped in many different ways, one of which is according to a fundamental aspect of audience analysis: their needs. Translation and communication processes usually aim to provide patients with biomedical knowledge about a specific health problem so that they can understand its basic aspects, such as symptoms, causes, risk factors, complications, diagnosis, treatment, prevention or prognosis of a specific disease. In this concept-based approach, the patient is a *knower* who needs to know these details to make a decision, as in the case of informed consent forms, or to perform a specific practical task such as taking a medicine safely and effectively, undergoing rehabilitation or following presurgery instructions.

A significant amount of patient-centred communication and translation is focused on performing specific tasks and achieving intended goals. Task analysis is the process of learning about ordinary users – in our case, patients. It is a useful way for writers and translators to test the quality of their work by performing the task that the addressees are supposed to do when or after reading the target text. In this task-oriented approach, the patient is a performer or *doer* who will need to be able to operationalise the information in the message. On other occasions, audiences need information to change their habits, from stopping smoking or using street drugs, to losing weight for medical reasons, to distancing themselves socially or wearing masks during a pandemic. In these cases, we can think of the audiences we are addressing as *behavers* in that messages will ideally have the impact of changing their behaviours. Finally, audiences can be addressed to share the experience of illness of individual patients, as in the case of patient narratives. Here the focus is on audiences as *experiencers* who have access to the real experiences of other patients (Figure 4.5).

- The knower – acquiring conceptual knowledge about relevant health issues
- The doer – applying knowledge to perform a task
- The behaver – achieving health-related behavioural changes
- The experiencer – aligning with the experience of other patients

FIGURE 4.5 General patient types according to their needs.

These four types should not be seen in isolation as exclusive categories but rather as dominant trends that often overlap. For example, doers, behavers and experiencers also need to be knowers, and behavers often need to perform specific tasks.

4.4.2 The challenge of patient diversity

In the clinical context, it is common to hear that there are as many types of patients as there are people, as everyone is unique and has different world views, life perspectives, personalities, and values (Beach & Inui 2006; Chalamon et al. 2013). In this section, we briefly discuss some of the main parameters for grouping patients: knowledge of the topic, attitudes towards the topic, audience size and demographics. These parameters can give rise to groupings as varied as paediatric patients, patients with limited health literacy, patients with chronic conditions, patients with disabilities, patients from LGTBQ+ communities, patients in emergency situations, patients with mental health issues, patients with limited language proficiency, cultural and ethnic language minority patients, elderly patients or patients at the end of life.

Knowledge of the topic

Topic is a key concept because it allows patients to be grouped on the basis of conceptual variables such as the disease they have, the symptoms they experience or the medication they take, to name but a few. In this way, communicators produce texts for specific groups of patients, for example with Parkinson's disease, with diabetes or with obesity or who take paracetamol.

Topics can vary widely. In fact, it is an open-ended category of analysis. Some topics are well established, while others are linked to cutting-edge research and require mediation processes to make them accessible and understandable to lay audiences, such as patients. The topic and content of the message are highly relevant aspects for communicators for producing reliable and accurate messages.

People's knowledge of a topic can vary widely, so communicators should find out what their audience already knows about it. Many chronic patients have accumulated information over the years and know a great deal about their condition. Other patients may be in the early stages and lack the background knowledge to understand some messages. Researching what the audience already knows about a medical or health topic can help to avoid both overestimating the audience's knowledge of the topic and drastically underestimating it, which risks sounding patronising.

Attitude towards health and illness

Patients can have very different attitudes towards health and illness: some are guided by a practical, utilitarian sense of health care, expecting only that their problems will be solved, while others give health care a more existential meaning linked to their psychological well-being. We also find patients – regardless of age, gender or culture – who want to play an active role in discussing all kinds of health issues with their doctor and take the initiative. Other patients prefer not to be informed or to delegate decisions to a family member. In addition, some patients display attitudes and behaviours that interfere with communication, such as aggressiveness, stubbornness, lack of motivation, dependence on the doctor or infantile behaviour. These make the task of health professionals more difficult (Pons 2006).

Some medical and health issues are ideologically and politically charged. Think of abortion or euthanasia. With diverse audiences, this can be problematic and requires careful consideration of how best to get the message across and which particular words we choose not to cause offence, trying to be as inclusive as possible.

Culture (see Chapter 1) also plays a crucial role in attitudes towards certain issues. There is a large body of academic literature on medical and health issues that are perceived differently across cultures. In the context of the Covid-19 pandemic, we witnessed the diversity of cultural and ideological attitudes towards social distancing, the use of masks in public spaces and vaccination. The attitudes of audiences in public and global health are particularly challenging.

Audience size

Audience size matters for writers, translators, interpreters and health professionals. The larger an audience is, the more diverse it can be in ideological, cultural, linguistic and accessibility terms, and the more communication challenges it will pose. Large audiences, such as those we address in public and global health, tend to be more multilingual and multicultural, requiring the use of translation into multiple languages, the use of multimodal solutions (see Chapter 3) to ensure access for all and the cultural adaptation of messages.

Demographics

The demographics of an audience include age, gender, religion, ethnic background, class, sexual orientation, occupation, education, group membership and countless other categories. Inclusiveness is a fundamental consideration. Using the mother tongue of the audience is the first step to achieving inclusiveness. Using the right register is also a must when addressing a diverse audience, for example in terms of age or educational background.

Figure 4.6 shows some common groupings by which patients and broader audiences can conceivably be categorised. However, communicators must be careful not to stereotype audiences based on demographic information; individuals are always more complicated than a simple identity category. For example, not all older people are intimidated by new technology and not all teenagers are only interested in social media.

- Language.
- Age. Writing or translating for an older audience is not the same as writing or translating for teenagers or children.
- Sex and gender. Breast cancer, menstruation, pregnancy risks, contraceptive advice, birth control and reproductive health are examples where patients of the same sex may be grouped together because they have common communication and information interests and needs.
- Culture. In many cases, cultural background can influence decision-making. Consider, for example, the Jehovah's Witnesses' ban on blood transfusions or the restrictions some religions place on the use of contraceptives.
- Knowledge of the subject.
- Attitude towards health and illness.
- Literacy level (often but not necessarily related to age) (see Chapter 5).
- Learning ability (see Chapter 3).
- Clinical characteristics: diagnosis, severity of illness, chronic vs non-chronic, co-morbidity, hypochondriac patients, "expert patients".

FIGURE 4.6 Diversity of patients according to different factors.

Suggestions for task. Analysing patients' attitudes

Collect the experiences of 10 people you know about their attitudes towards the health system (practical or existential) and whether they are involved in their therapeutic processes or prefer to delegate. Try to identify patterns and assess whether or not they can be related to age, literacy level, gender, etc.

4.5 Addressing your audience in a patient-centred way

Beyond specific genres and their accepted conventions in particular languages and contexts, in this final section, we summarise what might be called the common factors in addressing your audience in a patient-centred way (see Chapter 1).

When addressing your audience in a patient-centred way,

- Define your audience and its needs, purposes, expectations and circumstances (see Sections 4.2, 4.3 and 4.4).
- Consider the diversity of your audience. Audiences can be heterogeneous and have different sub-audiences (Sections 4.2 and 4.3). Depending on the breadth of your audience, you may need to produce more than one version of your document, bearing in mind potentially different languages and taboos. Informing adults about a particular condition will require a different strategy from that for informing children about the same condition. You may need to consider two or more audiences for the same communication.
- Consider different ways of reaching your audience, such as written texts, websites, apps, videos, podcasts or infographics (see Chapter 3). Consider using images, videos and diagrams to support the text.
- Address your audience in their mother tongue. Not being understood because of language barriers can be seen as care-related suffering. The more serious the illness, the more important it is to encourage patients to express themselves in their own language. Parkinson's disease, depression, autism and dementia are of particular interest because they can negatively affect speech and language use.
- Adapt your register, tenor and politeness to the characteristics of your audience. Avoid being too condescending.
- Communicate clearly and understandably. Optimise readability (see Chapter 5). Avoid jargon and unnecessary abstraction and use concrete images and language based on the patient's experience. Make it easy for patients to navigate by creating a coherent structure and using key words and phrases.
- Use storytelling where appropriate.
- Avoid institutionalised language that means nothing to patients.
- Treat your audience in a humane way. Avoid sexism, racism, ageism, ableism, homophobia, aporophobia (rejection of the poor), gerontophobia (rejection of the old) and other forms of prejudice against non-normative minorities. Use person-first language (see Chapter 6).

- Consider clearly stating the purpose of the document. Why is it important? What does the information mean to them in terms of their health and behaviour? Why should they care?
- Consider your audience when reviewing and revising your work. It is important to review the text through the eyes, ears and mind of the audience. Writing patient-centred texts requires us to put ourselves in the patient's shoes. For example, it is important to understand the cognitive and emotional challenges faced by patients who are elderly, impoverished or hopelessly ill.

Further reading

Hine, D. W.; Reser, J. P.; Morrison, M.; Phillips, W. J.; Nunn, P.; Cooksey, R. Audience Segmentation and Climate Change Communication: Conceptual and Methodological Considerations. *Wiley Interdisciplinary Reviews: Climate Change*, 2014, *5* (4), 441–459.

McQuail, D. *Audience Analysis*; Sage: London; New Delhi, 1997.

Moss, H. B.; Kirby, S. D.; Donodeo, F. Characterizing and Reaching High-Risk Drinkers Using Audience Segmentation. *Alcoholism: Clinical and Experimental Research*, 2009, *33* (8), 1336–1345.

Ommen, O.; Janssen, C.; Neugebauer, E.; Bouillon, B.; Rehm, K.; Rangger, C.; Pfaff, H. Trust, Social Support and Patient Type – Associations Between Patients Perceived Trust, Supportive Communication and Patients Preferences in Regard to Paternalism, Clarification and Participation of Severely Injured Patients. *Patient Education and Counseling*, 2008, *73* (2), 196–204.

Schmid, K. L.; Rivers, S. E.; Latimer, A. E.; Salovey, P. Targeting or Tailoring? Maximizing Resources to Create Effective Health Communications. *Marketing Health Services*, 2008, *28* (1), 32.

Slater, M. D. Theory and Method in Health Audience Segmentation. *Journal of Health Communication*, 1996, *1* (3), 267–284.

Stand Up, Speak Out: The Practice and Ethics of Public Speaking. https://saylordotorg.github.io/text_stand-up-speak-out-the-practice-and-ethics-of-public-speaking/s08-audience-analysis.html

Strekalova, Y. A. Seekers and Avoiders: Using Health Information Orientation to Explore Audience Segmentation. *Journal of Communication in Healthcare*, 2014, *7* (3), 228–237.

5

CREATING TEXTS FOR PATIENTS

Comprehensibility

Overview of chapter

Comprehensibility is a concept that applies to any kind of communication (oral, written, multimodal), and it is a particularly sensitive issue in patient-centred translation and writing. It has become increasingly important for patients and the general public to understand information relating to their health. This chapter focuses on the lack of comprehensibility in texts intended for patients, which can be a major obstacle to patient compliance and thus to the effectiveness of health care systems.

The first area we address is comprehensibility (Section 5.1). Information for patients has traditionally been designed and delivered from the point of view of the health professional, often ignoring the needs and expectations of the final reader, the patient. Comprehensibility is not easy to define, but we contend that it refers to the sum of elements that allow patients to understand the text adequately. Comprehensibility has mainly to do with the conceptual complexity of content. However, we need to consider some additional aspects such as format, typographical legibility, linguistic readability and colour and image.

The second area we deal with is the need to improve texts for patients to correct their lack of comprehensibility, as shown in a large number of studies and reported by organisations such as the WHO (Section 5.2). Most analyses only use quantitative criteria and tools to measure the comprehensibility of texts – the so-called *readability formulas* – and propose solutions for writing and translating texts based on these purely numerical approaches. We argue that eluding qualitative approaches that take into account the patient's perspective to measure and improve comprehensibility can lead to incomplete

DOI: 10.4324/9780429299698-6

and misleading interpretations. To improve the comprehensibility of texts, there are simplification strategies including using plain language, synthesising information and simplifying medical terms (Section 5.3).

5.1 Defining and characterising comprehesibility

After a series of consultations for a rectal bleeding problem caused by internal haemorrhoids, the doctor determined that Olivia's problem could not be resolved with the medication she had been prescribed and that a small surgical intervention was necessary. As she left the consultation, the nurse gave her a document and explained that it was a consent form to be signed on the day of the operation. Upon returning home, Olivia carefully reviewed the document, which was meant to help her decide whether or not to agree to the planned procedure. However, she did not understand the technical information about the procedure or what the consequences of not signing it would have. Therefore, Olivia returned to the hospital to seek clarification from the nurse who had given her the consent form. Regrettably, the nurse played down the content and advised her to simply sign it, a common practice among patients, even if they do not understand the content, as consent is typically a prerequisite for any medical intervention.

As previously mentioned, Olivia is a curious patient and was not satisfied with the response. She could have turned to the internet to find out more but realised that it was a delicate situation. She was concerned about the possibility of not finding reliable information to help her make a decision and did not want to expose herself to potential misinformation, contrary to what is usually the case. Consequently, she requested a meeting with her doctor to gain understanding of the document and finally signed it with confidence only after the doctor explained the aspects she found confusing.

Olivia's struggle to understand the information she was provided with is at the heart of many barriers in patient-centred translation and communication. We argue that the problem is not Olivia herself but the quality of the information she has been given. In particular, we think that the information is not comprehensible enough.

Defining comprehensibility is challenging. Following Jensen (2015: 166), *comprehensibility* is "the lowest possible textual complexity". Dale and Chall (1949) define comprehensibility from the perspective of the readers' experience: "The total sum (including all the interactions) of all those elements (legibility, interest, and ease of understanding) within a given piece of printed material that affect the success a group of readers have with it". For them, success refers to the extent to which readers understand texts, read them at an optimal speed and find them interesting. For Dubay (2004: 3) "readability is what makes some texts easier to read than others. It is often confused with legibility, which concerns type face and layout."

In our view, we need to combine the concepts of *readability* and *legibility* under the more general notion of comprehensibility, which covers all the linguistic, typographical and content-related features of texts and how they affect the ways patients receive and perceive them (García-Izquierdo & Montalt 2017). Comprehensibility is not restricted to a specific target audience, such as patients as lay audiences. Something can be considered comprehensible even if it requires some background knowledge or effort to understand, as in the case of expert readers. In the case of comprehensibility focused on patients, the notion of lay friendliness (Jensen & Zethsen 2012) refers to the quality of being easily understood by someone who does not have specialised knowledge or training in a particular subject. It emphasises clarity, simplicity and avoidance of jargon or complex concepts. Something considered lay friendly should be readily understandable by the average person.

Researchers in the fields of health communication, applied linguistics and translation are unanimous in stressing the paramount importance of ensuring comprehensibility in texts intended for patients. Although this may seem self-evident, patient information has historically been produced and disseminated primarily from the perspective of health professionals, often neglecting the needs and expectations of the ultimate reader: the individual patient.

Since the 1990s, with the institutionalisation of research ethics and the expansion of science education, there has been a growing emphasis on the importance of ensuring that citizens, users, clients and patients can understand health-related information. This shift is further underscored by recommendations from organisations such as the WHO and health authority ethics committees in the US and Europe. These bodies advocate the consideration of patients' needs and expectations in the context of patient-centred care to ensure that health information is understandable.

There is widespread agreement that the effectiveness of a treatment or therapeutic procedure depends largely on the patient's understanding of the information provided. Medical organisations have noted numerous complaints from users that suggest that the lack of comprehension results from a failure to adopt a functionalist view of comprehensibility. According to this view, texts should serve a specific function and be tailored to the needs of the reader. As Jensen (2015) emphasises, comprehensibility should not be seen as an inherent quality of the text alone but must also take into account the context, including the characteristics and circumstances of the reader.

Comprehensibility refers to the ease or difficulty with which readers can understand a text (Wolfer 2015), a factor influenced by their level of literacy and how communicators address them. Literacy is not a single characteristic but rather a spectrum that includes different levels and corresponding abilities. When translating or writing medical texts, it's crucial to consider how patients understand the information presented. They should also be aware of the different strategies available to tailor their communication to the needs of their target audience. A key point emphasised in this chapter is the considerable variability in patients' literacy levels and the importance of adapting communication strategies accordingly.

In a health culture that relies heavily on written information, literacy plays a crucial role in understanding another important concept discussed in this chapter: health literacy (Pilegaard & Havn 2012). Coined in the USA in the 1970s, health literacy refers to the extent to which individuals have the ability to obtain, process and understand basic health information and services needed to make appropriate health decisions (Institute of Medicine 2004). According to Smith et al. (2018), health literacy is increasingly recognised as an independent determinant of health-related outcomes. Since the 1970s, numerous national and international initiatives have focused on researching and promoting literacy and health literacy, including the National Assessment of Adult Literacy in the USA or the European Health Literacy Survey (Hansvberry et al. 2013).

Overall, it's reasonable to assume that patients with lower literacy are likely to have lower health literacy, particularly in health systems where key information is predominantly presented in written form. Risk factors associated with low health literacy include older age, belonging to a racial minority, limited education, low socioeconomic status and belonging to a linguistic minority. However, a paradox may arise for migrant patients: they may have high literacy in their home health care culture but face language-related challenges in accessing health care in the host country.

Comprehensible information plays a crucial role in improving patients' health literacy, enabling them to understand and engage effectively with health-related content. Health literacy, in turn, facilitates comprehensibility by enabling individuals to interpret and critically appraise health information, navigate the health care system and make informed decisions about their health. Strategies such as providing information in plain language and using visual aids help to improve comprehension and promote health literacy. This mutually reinforcing relationship highlights the importance of promoting both understandable information and health literacy to empower patients and improve health outcomes.

5.1.1 Factors that determine comprehensibility

The factors that can determine the level of comprehensibility of a text are:

- **Contents.** Degree of terminological density in texts and organisation of content into themes and sequences to form a structure; use of rhetorical moves depending on textual typology or predominant function of every part of the text (Hatim & Mason 1990; Göpferich 2009) (e.g. exposition, argumentation, instruction).

- **Linguistic readability.** Grammatical construction (active vs. passive voice; simple vs. complex sentences), vocabulary and expressions.
- **Typographical legibility.** Type and font size, use of margins and contrast between lettering and background.
- **Format.** Dimensions (number and size of pages, if on paper, or amount of scrolling on websites), quality of paper or quality of the medium in multimodal presentations.
- **Colour and images.** Graphs, illustrations, photographs, infographics.

Text comprehensibility cannot be attributed solely to qualities inherent in the text itself but is deeply intertwined with contextual factors and the characteristics of the readers. While some texts may appear straightforward and easily understandable to some readers, they may pose significant challenges to others, and factors such as the reader's literacy level, cultural background, language skills, cognitive abilities and prior knowledge play crucial roles in how comprehensible a text is perceived to be. In addition, the context in which the text is presented – including the purpose of communication, the medium used, cultural norms and the specific communicative situation – can have a significant impact on its comprehensibility.

For example, a medical document written in technical language may be understandable to health professionals but difficult for patients with limited health literacy. Therefore, to fully understand and assess the comprehensibility of a text, it is essential to consider the complex interplay between textual features, contextual factors and the characteristics of the readers. By recognising the dynamic nature of comprehensibility, communicators can effectively tailor their messages to ensure that they resonate with their intended audience and achieve their communication goals.

The consideration of texts with different levels of difficulty is essential due to the existence of different patient typologies, as discussed in Chapter 4. For example, communicating information to children requires a different approach from what's needed to communicate with adults. In addition, the adult population has a wide range of literacy levels and formal educational backgrounds, ranging from expert patients to those who are virtually illiterate. There are also differences in how people approach discussing health issues, with some being open and others preferring euphemisms, especially around sensitive topics such as sexuality, excretory function or death. In addition, migrant populations face language challenges. It is therefore crucial to tailor information to these different levels of complexity.

5.1.2 Lack of comprehensibility

The WHO and many researchers in the fields of medicine and applied linguistics and translation highlight the lack of comprehensibility of texts addressed to patients, both in terms of typographical legibility (inappropriate format and presentation) and in terms of the difficulty in understanding the information they contain (linguistic legibility) (García-Izquierdo & Montalt 2017; Sivanadarajah et al. 2017; Ribeiro-Alves & Ferreira Cabrera 2018). The causes can include failure to consider lack of background knowledge, poor organization, inaccessible language, sentence structure, ambiguity and use of medical terminology without explanation.

Numerous studies, readily available through databases such as Medline/PubMed, provide compelling evidence of the detrimental impact of poor comprehension on various aspects of patient outcomes and health care delivery. For example, research has consistently shown that patients who have difficulty understanding health-related information are more likely to have difficulty adhering to prescribed treatments and medication regimens. In specialties such as cardiology and endocrinology, where patients may require ongoing monitoring and management of complex conditions such as heart disease or diabetes, poor understanding can lead to missed appointments, inappropriate self-management practices and increased risk of complications. Similarly, in surgical specialties, inadequate understanding of preoperative instructions or postoperative care can lead to surgical complications, prolonged recovery times and dissatisfaction with treatment outcomes.

This lack of comprehensibility can lead to suboptimal health outcomes, increased hospitalisations and higher health care costs. In addition, poor comprehension can have significant impacts on patient satisfaction, as individuals may feel frustrated or dissatisfied if they have difficulty understanding medical instructions or explanations provided by health care providers. Poor comprehension can also impede effective communication between patients and health care professionals, hindering the exchange of important information, shared decision-making and ultimately the quality of care that patients receive.

Collectively, these studies highlight the urgent need to prioritise efforts to improve the comprehensibility of health-related information in order to improve patient adherence, satisfaction and overall health outcomes. Overall, while some researchers focus on identifying the challenges associated with poor comprehensibility, others actively seek to develop and evaluate practical solutions and interventions to improve patient understanding and promote better health outcomes. By proactively addressing comprehensibility issues and implementing evidence-based interventions, health care providers and policy makers can work towards improving patient-centred care and reducing health inequalities.

Every patient is unique, making it a challenge to meet all their expectations. There's often a disconnect between what the health care industry and clinicians assume patients want and the reality of patient preferences, particularly when it comes to being involved in their own health care decisions. However, current guidelines recognise the growing importance of patient engagement due to evolving regulations and a commitment to transparency. There's a need to present health care data and messages in a way that is understandable and useful to the general public. Achieving this is a significant challenge and requires a distinct set of medical writing skills tailored to lay audiences, as opposed to the approach used for regulatory purposes.

In the context of multiculturalism and pluralism in health care, the relationship between the formal and the conceptual complexity of texts is not always straightforward. On the one hand, there are texts that may appear accessible or conceptually simple but their presentation may be complicated by the stylistic choices of the author or translator or because they are written by experts in the field who use specialised discursive conventions that may not conform to standard language usage. On the other hand, there are texts that may appear simple in form but contain culturally specific references or alternative worldviews, such as religious or alternative medicine texts, which introduce conceptual complexities that require interpretation. This underlines the importance of comprehensibility, a consideration crucial for medical translators and writers who must navigate these complexities in order to communicate effectively with diverse audiences.

5.2 Assessing comprehensibility

Assessing comprehensibility often requires a combination of quantitative measures and qualitative judgements based on actual reader feedback. Factors such as clarity, organisation, coherence and the audience's familiarity with the subject matter all play a role in determining how easy it is to understand a piece of text.

5.2.1 Readability formulas

The use of readability formulas, such as those of Flesch, Dale, Chall, SMOG, and FORCAST, dates back to the 1920s. Readability makes some texts easier to read than others (Jarret & Redish 2019). These formulas, in general, analyse the number of sentences statistically, sentence length per 100 periods (because shorter sentences increase readability), number of (different) words per sentence (a common plain English guideline prescribes an average of 15–20 words), word length (because, for example, Graeco-Latin terminology tends to use longer words, which can add complexity to the text), number of sentences per paragraph, vocabulary frequency lists (because vocabulary has an important role in readability as a predictor of text difficulty), grade level of reading difficulty (the same text will be easier for those with higher-grade-level reading skills than for those with less advanced skills) (Jarret & Redish 2019).

The Flesch Reading Ease scale, created by Rudolf Flesch, is one of the most frequently used formulas (Flesch 1949; Table 5.1).

TABLE 5.1 Flesch's Reading Ease scores

Reading Ease Score	*Style Description*	*Estimated Reading Grade*	*Estimated Percent of US Adults (1949)*
0 to 30:	Very Difficult	College graduate	4.5
30 to 40:	Difficult	13th to 16th grade	33
50 to 60:	Fairly Difficult	10th to 12th grade	54
60 to 70:	Standard	8th and 9th grade	83
70 to 80:	Fairly Easy	7th grade	88
80 to 90:	Easy	6th grade	91
90 to 100:	Very Easy	5th grade	93

Flesch's Reading Ease formula has become the most widely used, tested. and reliable (Chall 1958; Klare 1963). To further simplify the Flesch Reading Ease formula, Farr et al. (1951) substituted the average number of one-syllable words. More recently, Szigriszt (1993) validated the Flesch Reading Ease Formula in his PhD thesis in developing the Flesch-Szigriszt index, Inflesz. The Inflesz index has five degrees of difficulty:

<40 Very difficult. University, scientific texts
40–55 Somewhat difficult. High school texts, popularizing magazines, specialised press
55–65 Normal. Secondary school texts, general press, sports press
65–80 Quite easy. Primary education texts, popularizing novels, tabloids
>80 Very easy. Primary education texts. Comics, for example.

The reading grade for a text depends on its usage; the same text will be easier for those with more advanced reading skills.

Some European countries have their own versions of readability indices, in most cases, adaptations of the Inflesz formula. For instance, in Italy, the Vacca Model of 1972 and the Gulpease Index of 1988 established three levels of education – elementary, intermediate, higher – based on word lengths. In France, the Scolarius website combines different formulas and text types to indicate suitability to readers' educational levels. In Germany, the Wiener Sachtextformel by Richard Bamberger and Erich Valeck addresses the challenge of German's typically very long words and sentences (see some tools for measuring text readability in Task 5.1). Over the course of almost a century, readability formulas have gradually improved. This evolution includes a study of the structural characteristics of the text, such as prepositional phrases and indeterminate clauses.

5.2.2 *Beyond the limitations of quantitative measurements*

In the 1970s, efforts were made to measure other features related to content, organisation, coherence and the design of texts. However, these formulas still have limitations. In spite of the success of the readability formulas, they were always the centre of controversy (Dubay 2004: 2).

The readability of text is often measured using different formulas and computer programs. However, these methods can produce different results due to differences in the way they count linguistic elements such as sentences, words or syllables. Factors such as which aspects of language are prioritised and the algorithms used can contribute to these discrepancies. Therefore, while the usefulness of such formulas should not be dismissed, as they have contributed significantly to the analysis of literacy and text comprehension and difficulty, it is important to expand the analysis to include qualitative research that focuses on the needs of patients as readers of the texts (García-Izquierdo & Montalt 2017).

Hence, quantitative and numerical research using readability formulas can lead to incomplete and misleading interpretations of text comprehensibility. Patient studies, as shown by Munsour et al. (2017), demonstrate that even in texts with seemingly low or moderate levels of complexity, in terms of formulas, patients can consider that some elements do not meet their expectations. For instance, lexical choices might offend sensibilities, tend towards impersonality or reflect a lack of empathy (see Chapter 6). Therefore, we believe it is important to complement the formulaic results with qualitative analyses of the texts conducted by linguistic and translation specialists, as well as by medical professionals and patients. In other words, all the individuals involved in the process must provide their opinions on the final result, particularly patients (see Chapter 7).

TASK 5.1 CRITICAL COMMENT ON THE USEFULNESS OF READABILITY FORMULAS FOR IMPROVING THE COMPREHENSIBILITY

Materials

Tools for measuring text readability:

www.wyliecomm.com/2021/01/measure-readability-with-these-5-readability-apps/https://readabilityformulae.com/free-readability-formula-tests.php
https://readable.com/
www.online-utility.org/english/readability_test_and_improve.jsp

Texts:

MSD Manual Professional Version (http://www.msdmanuals.com/professional)
MSD Manual Consumer Version ((http://www.msdmanuals.com/home)

Procedure

1) Select an excerpt from the MSD Manual Professional Version in a language of your choice. Use one of the readability tests proposed to analyse it.
2) Carefully analyse the information obtained from applying the test. Rewrite the list of sentences that the program suggests you need to consider re-writing to improve readability and introduce your proposal in the analyser again to see if it effectively improves the results.
3) Compare your version with the consumer version of the same excerpt provided in the MSD Manual Consumer Version.

5.3 Some recommendations to improve comprehensibility

In order to improve comprehensibility and contribute to bridging the gap between two different knowledge and discourse communities, namely health professionals and patients, specialised medical information needs to be adequately recontextualized, that is, "move[d] to a target context with different participants, purposes, expectations, values, etc.", and reformulated, which involves "a textual operation of rearranging and reexpressing the content in a different target text" (Montalt & Shuttleworth 2012: 16).

Within translation studies, intralingual translation (Jakobson 1959/2000; Zethsen 2009) and expert-lay translation (Zethsen 2007, 2018) are conceptual frameworks that prove useful for making texts more patient-friendly and improving comprehensibility, as they involve rewriting, recontextualising and reformulating information in the same language to adapt it to a lay reader's needs. This rewriting process generally involves a *genre shift* (Montalt & González 2007), which means transforming a specialised genre (e.g. a research article) into one addressed to the general public (e.g. a summary for patients). Genre shift is particularly useful because it helps to "bridge the gap between the patient's right to know and the patient's ability to understand and guarantees the continuity of communication between different expertise communities" (Ezpeleta 2012: 175).

An increasing number of genres written for specialists are currently being intralingually translated to meet the needs of non-specialist audiences. We can find examples in the fact sheets for patients published by the European Society for Medical Oncology, which derive from clinical practice guidelines – a genre aimed at medical professionals based on a systematic review of clinical evidence to support decision-making processes in patient care. The consumer version provided online by the prestigious MSD Manual, where content related to diseases, diagnostic procedures or health news is explained so that the general public can understand it, is another example in which genre shifts or intralingual translation are carried out (see Chapter 2).

We can also find an increasing number of portals and webpages about medicine and health that are specifically addressed to patients and the general public, such as *Familydoctor.org, Saludalia* and *PatientsUpToDate*. Apart from explaining medical information in a way a lay reader can understand it, they include other elements that enhance comprehensibility, such as infographics, photographs, drawings and links to other sites. Some websites even offer users the option to select information tailored to their level of education and their specific needs.

5.3.1 Some strategies for improving comprehensibility of texts addressed to patients

The strategies used when performing intralingual translations and genre shifts are particularly useful for health professionals, translators and writers to improve both the legibility and comprehensibility of texts addressed to patients. These strategies are varied and affect the text on both the macrotextual (content, structure and organization of information) and the microtextual (morpho-syntactic and lexical mechanisms) levels: for example, it is often important for a lay reader to know the agent of the sentence, so the use of the active voice and verbs instead of nouns usually help the lay reader to understand the medical content better. It is also generally advisable to break up long sentences up and organise the information they contain in a logical and easy-to-understand way.

Information that is not relevant to a lay audience should be omitted, but it goes without saying that the medical expert author of the text to be translated or adapted should be consulted before anything is omitted. In addition, lay audiences often lack background knowledge that specialist audiences have or are assumed to have, so it is often necessary to make this knowledge explicit in the target text in order to help the reader understand it. Changes in the structure of information should also be considered to create a sequence that is relevant to the target reader. Pictograms and other visual aids may be needed in the target text.

Strategies that help to clarify the terminology, which is "the most obvious barrier" (Ciapuscio 2003: 222), are particularly relevant when addressing the reader in a comprehensive way. These determinologisation strategies include synonymy, explanation, definition, exemplification, illustration, analogy, comparison and using more popular terms (Campos Andrés 2013). Metaphors can also play an important role, since "complex and more abstract areas of science rely particularly on metaphor and analogy to add clarity to knowledge and to communicate that knowledge" (Braithwaite et al. 2006).

Table 5.2 summarises procedures for improving readability at both macrotextual and microtextual levels. At the macrotextual level, it suggests

TABLE 5.2 Strategies for improving comprehensibility

Level	*Aspect affected*	*Procedures to be used*
Macrotextual	General structure	• Restructuring the overall text; shortening paragraphs
	Content	• Selecting only the most relevant information • Adding background information not found in the original and making relevant information explicit
	Typography, layout and visual support	• Incorporating visual elements (figures, illustrations and tables) • Using vertical numbered or bulleted lists • Avoiding capital letters • Emphasizing keywords • Avoiding justification, hyphenation and footnotes
Microtextual (Morphosyntax)	Sentence structure	• Shortening sentences; simplifying syntax
	Verbs	• Preferring transitive verbs and simple tenses
	Voice	• Using the active voice
	Noun phrases	• Replacing noun phrases by verbal clauses.
	Tenor	• Addressing the reader directly
	Punctuation marks	• Increasing the number of punctuation marks to introduce explanations, definitions, etc.
Microtextual (Lexis)	Technical terms or concepts	• Keeping the technical term and adding explanations/metaphors/comparisons/ exemplifications • Eliminating the technical term and replacing it with equivalents/ explanations/paraphrases • Rewording abstract concepts in a nonabstract manner • Using redundancy techniques (repetitions, synonyms) for complex concepts • Translating officialese into lay vocabulary

Source: adapted from Muñoz-Miquel (2012) and Zethsen & Montalt (2022)

restructuring the text, selecting relevant content and incorporating visual elements. Microtextual adjustments include simplifying sentence structure, favouring active voice, and clarifying technical terms. These strategies aim to improve comprehension and accessibility for readers.

In order to effectively implement comprehensibility strategies, it's essential to actively involve the intended audience. By engaging with the audience, whether through usability testing, focus groups or surveys (see Chapter 7), we can gain valuable insights into their needs, preferences and comprehension levels. This collaborative approach ensures that the adjustments made to the text are closely aligned with the audience's expectations and understanding, ultimately increasing the effectiveness of the communication.

A collaborative approach to patient-centred translation and communication should be based on co-creation. This process involves the active engagement of patients, carers, health care providers and language experts in the development and refinement of communication materials. The aim is to ensure that the information provided is clear, culturally sensitive and tailored to the needs and preferences of the target audience. By incorporating feedback from different stakeholders, we strive to create communication materials that are accessible, accurate and respectful of patients' backgrounds and needs.

TASK 5.2 EXPLORING COMPREHENSIBILITY: SIMPLIFYING TERMINOLOGY

Materials

MSD Manual Professional Version (http://www.msdmanuals/professional)
MSD Manual Consumer Version (http://www.msdmanuals/home)

Procedure

1) Select a topic from the MSD Manual Professional Version and the MSD Manual Consumer Version in a language of your choice.
2) Read the texts carefully and try to detect differences in aspects such as simplifying language (definitions, paraphrases, synonymy, etc.) and improving linguistic readability, taking into account the recommendations in this chapter.

TASK 5.3 EXPLORING COMPREHENSIBILITY: CLEAR STRUCTURE (TEXTUAL TYPOLOGY AND RHETORICAL MOVES)

Materials

Fact sheets for patients in Spanish and English

(www.reproductivefacts.org/news-and-publications/patient-fact-sheets-and-booklets/documents/fact-sheets-and-info-booklets-en-espanol/)

Informed consent

(https://clinicaltrials.gov/ProvidedDocs/02/NCT03319602/ICF_000.pdf)

Procedure

Try to determine which type of rhetorical sequence (move) and which textual typology (expository, argumentative or instructive) predominates in the fact sheet and informed consent texts and consider whether the language is appropriate for conveying the information for the average reader. Justify your answer.

TASK 5.4 EXPLORING GENRE SHIFTS

Materials

Consider this summary for patients on bone marrow transplants, published in *Annals of Internal Medicine*. Consult the original research article it comes from at www.ncbi.nlm.nih.gov/pmc/articles/PMC7847247/.

Summaries for Patients February 18, 2020

Patient Outcomes After Bone Marrow Transplant

What is the problem and what is known about it so far?

When cancer does not respond adequately to standard doses of chemotherapy or radiation, higher doses might be more effective. But high-dose chemotherapy and radiation can be highly toxic to the bone marrow, where normal blood cells are made. The toxic effects can be managed by using blood-forming cells donated by another person to replenish the patient's bone marrow. The donor cells can also eliminate cancer cells. Ten years ago, researchers at a center that specializes in this kind of therapy reported that outcomes had been improving for patients having transplants using donor cells, although many patients continued to have dangerous or even deadly complications.

Why did the researchers do this particular study?

To find out whether outcomes have continued to improve since the prior report for patients having transplants using donor cells, despite older and sicker patients now coming for transplant.

Who was studied?

All patients who had a transplant using donor cells at the researchers' center between 2003 and 2007 and between 2013 and 2017.

How was the study done?

The researchers collected information on the patients to see if complication rates and survival had changed.

What did the researchers find?

Rates of transplant complications improved compared with those in the earlier period. Rates of infectious, gastrointestinal, kidney, and respiratory complications had decreased, and in some cases, the complications that did occur were less severe overall. Survival also improved, although death due to inability to cure the cancer remains a major problem.

What were the limitations of the study?

The study included patients treated at only 1 expert medical center, and the results might not be the same among patients treated at other centers.

What are the implications of the study?

Treatment and outcomes for patients having transplants using donor cells have continued to improve, although the challenge of further decreasing rates of complications and cancer recurrence remains.

Procedure

Consider whether the language used differs sufficiently from that of the research article it comes from and fulfils the purpose of the genre. Pay attention to the micro- and macro-textual levels proposed in the Table 5.2.

Further reading

Arévalos Ramírez, R. E.; Martínez-Mercado, A.; Vera Almirón, Y. G.; Báez Larrea, N. D.; Báez Larrea, N. F.; Paniagua Cristaldo, D. R. Linguistic Legibility of Printed Informational Materials, Disclosed by the Ministry of Public Health and Social Welfare, Paraguay, Applying the Gunning Fog Index. *Revista de salud pública del Paraguay*, 2019, *9* (2), 53–57.

Barrio Cantalejo, I. El Programa INFLESZ. *Legibilidad.com*. Una web sobre el análisis de la legibilidad de textos escritos en español, 2015. http://legibilidad.blogspot.com

Brøgger, M. N.; Zethsen, K. K. Inter-and Intralingual Translation of Medical Information: The Importance of Comprehensibility. In *The Routledge Handbook of Translation and Health*; Routledge, 2021; pp. 96–107.

Friedman, D. B.; Hoffman-Goetz, L. A Systematic Review of Readability and Comprehension Instruments Used for Print and Web-Based Cancer Information. *Health Education & Behavior*, 2006, *33* (3), 352–373.

Hill-Madsen, A. Lexical Strategies in Intralingual Translation between Registers. *Hermes*, 2015, *54*, 85–105. Electronic Version. https://tidsskrift.dk/index.php/her/article/view/22949/20059.

López-Picazo, J. J.; Tomás-Garcia, N.; Abellán, M. R. ¿Pero alguien entiende los consentimientos informados? Una propuesta para facilitar su comprensión. *Revista de Calidad Asistencial*, 2016, *31* (4), 182–189.

Muñoz Miquel, A.; Ezpeleta, P.; Saiz-Hontangas, P. Intralingual Translation in Healthcare Settings: Strategies and Proposals for Medical Translator Training. *MONTI*, 2018, *10*, 177–204.

Stossel, L. M.; Segar, N.; Gliatto, P.; Fallar, R.; Karani, R. Readability of Patient Education Materials Available at the Point of Care. *Journal of General Internal Medicine*, 2012, *27* (9), 1165–1170. https://doi.org/10.1007/s11606-012-2046-0.

Zethsen, K. K. Intralingual Translation. *Handbook of Translation Studies*, 2021, *5*, 135–142.

6

CREATING TEXTS FOR PATIENTS

Empathy

Overview of chapter

Together with comprehensibility, empathy is perhaps the most important determining factor for successful patient-centred communication in clinical settings. Behaving empathetically means aligning with, and understanding the feelings, thoughts and attitudes of, the other person, that is, the ability to put oneself in another person's shoes, if only to a limited extent. Patient-centred communication aims to share health information in a clear, compassionate and emotionally supportive way. This chapter focuses on empathy and how to show and foster it, both orally and in writing.

The first aspect we address is how we understand empathy within the paradigm of patient-centred communication (Section 6.1). We emphasise the growing recognition of the power of empathic communication to promote healing, reduce suffering, empower patients, increase patients' satisfaction and adherence, reduce anxiety and distress and improve health outcomes. The second area is empathy in oral communication (Section 6.2). Many recent empirical studies point out the need for empathetic face-to-face patient–doctor interactions in the consultation. Parameters of empathy (e.g. eye contact, active listening, tone of voice, body language) as well as examples of strategies for building empathy in face-to-face interactions are dealt with.

The third theme is how to convey empathy in written texts (Section 6.3). Empathy in face-to-face interactions can be conveyed through many non-verbal elements which cannot be present in written texts. However, in written texts, other empathetic strategies can be effectively employed such as personalising information, adjusting tenor, using plain language and simplifying technical terms. Finally, in the last section, we explore some aspects regarding cultural

DOI: 10.4324/9780429299698-7

variation in the expression of empathy (Section 6.4). What is perfectly polite and acceptable in one language may not evoke the same reaction in another. Ways of making requests or giving advice to patients in English will probably differ from how the same functions are usually expressed in other languages. Degrees of explicitness and directness – for example, when referring to different parts of the body – may also differ culturally and linguistically.

6.1 What is empathy?

Throughout our lives, we have probably visited different health care providers, either as patients or as accompanying persons. In those consultations, we may have encountered health professionals who just looked at the computer screen and did not listen to us, or who did not let us explain ourselves or ask questions when we needed to. We may also have experienced situations in which the complete opposite happened: despite receiving a bad diagnosis during the consultation, we went home relieved, because we felt listened to, comforted by a look or a gesture, and satisfied because we were able to openly discuss all our doubts with the physician.

During her therapeutic process as a patient, Olivia, after receiving an informed consent form that she did not understand properly, went back to the consultation for clarification and she found that the doctor was able to align with her and provided her with the information she needed in an empathic way. We intuitively know what empathy (and the lack of it) is and how we notice it. But how can we define empathy? Is it a natural, inborn human quality or an ability that can – or must – be either acquired or formally learned later in life? What makes communication truly empathic?

The concept of empathy has been approached from different fields of knowledge, such as psychology, education or biology. Even neuroscience has dealt with empathy, with significant progresses achieved in establishing its neurological basis thanks to the discovering of the mirror neuron system. Generally speaking, empathy is referred to as the ability to recognise and understand the thoughts and feelings of another person and respond to them (Edlins & Dolamore 2018). It involves aligning into another person's point of view, rather than just one's own, and is crucial for establishing rapport in relationships. In this regard, a distinction should be made between *sympathy, empathy* and *compassion*. These terms are often used interchangeably, because they are closely related, but they refer to slightly different concepts.

Sympathy and empathy both involve a caring response to the emotional state of another person. Sympathy is a feeling of authentic concern for someone who is experiencing something difficult or painful and a desire that they become better off, while empathy also implies actively sharing in the emotional experience of the other person rather than just feeling bad for them.

Compassion and empathy refer to a caring response to someone else's distress, but compassion adds to that emotional experience a desire to alleviate the person's distress and even to act on that person's behalf.

In health care settings, empathy – also referred to as alignment or being aligned with the patient – has been defined as "the competence of a health professional to understand the patient's situation, perspective, and feelings; to communicate that understanding and check its accuracy; and to act on that understanding in a helpful therapeutic way" (Derksen et al. 2013: e76). In patient-centred care, it is recognised that messages convey not only content but also emotions, attitudes, status, norms of interaction and expectations (Du Pré & Foster 2015). Thus, empathy becomes a basic component of the therapeutic relationship and is even identified as the core of caring (Ruiz-Moral et al. 2017).

From the perspective of the health sciences; social psychology; cultural anthropology and applied linguistics, translation and interpreting studies, there is growing recognition of the power of empathic communication to promote healing, reduce suffering, empower patients, increase patients' satisfaction and adherence, reduce anxiety and distress and improve health outcomes (Brown et al. 2015; Montalt & García-Izquierdo 2016). Evidence from outpatients strongly indicates that when doctors respond to patients' emotions and distress, patient satisfaction increases (Kalavana 2015). This is why most patients would recommend an empathic physician over one who is not (Vedsted & Heje 2008). Empathy is also a value that is expected to be offered by workers in public services (Valero Garcés & Alcalde Peñalver 2021).

6.1.1 Empathy in patient-centred communication

Six core functions of patient-doctor interaction are of key importance in patient centred communication and can be achieved by means of both verbal and non-verbal strategies (Epstein & Street 2007; Dean & Street 2015):

1) Fostering healing relationships: enhancing trust and rapport.
2) Exchanging information: ensuring that patients understand it and that their needs and preferences are met.
3) Responding to emotions: identifying direct and indirect emotional cues and addressing them with empathy and warmth.
4) Managing uncertainty: helping patients cope with uncertainty and mitigating their fears while maintaining a balance between truth and hope.
5) Making decisions: providing information, offering opportunities for involvement, encouraging participation and accommodating patients' preferences.
6) Enabling patient empowerment and self-management: providing autonomy-supportive behaviours, guidance and access to resources.

These functions are not independent of one another and often overlap. Although there is a specific function (responding to emotions) in which empathy plays a key role, it can be said to be common to all of them. Empathy involves three dimensions, according to Du Pré and Foster (2015): paying attention to another person's emotions (relational), understanding those emotions (cognitive) and responding to those emotions (communicative). Therefore, empathy is also required to build healing relationships, to be able to detect when patients do not understand medical information and tailor the way in which it is delivered and to help them make decisions and manage uncertainty. Empathy is thus an integrative practice rather than an individual skill in medical communication (Marsden 2014). In multilingual health care settings – where health professionals and patients may not share the same language –, the patient's mother tongue is a crucial factor.

Some medical fields are particularly prone to cognitive complexity and emotional intensity and therefore require more sensitivity and empathy on the part of health professionals. Palliative care, oncology, infertility and mental health are just a few examples of specialties in which empathy is crucial. Unfortunately, many study findings show that medical professionals, even in these specialities, often remain neutral and restrict themselves to providing accurate factual information (Gustin et al. 2015); when patients express emotional cues, either overtly or covertly, in medical consultations, doctors tend to avoid such communication and focus on the medical content instead of recognising those cues and responding with empathy (Kalavana 2015; Du Pré & Foster 2015). The question is: Do they avoid it because they do not want to respond to those emotional cues or because they do not know how to listen actively and respond to them?

One of the problems behind this situation is that empathy has traditionally been considered intuitive and unteachable (Silverman 2015), a matter of personality, as patients themselves suggest (García-Izquierdo & Muñoz-Miquel 2015). In fact, the most critical issue for medical students is how to deal with emotion (Hausberg et al. 2012), since skills in this area can be poor and difficult to develop. There is also strong evidence that empathy declines as medical students enter their final years of training (Kalavana 2015). Recent studies carried out by the GENTT Group at the Universitat Jaume I in Spain (Bellés-Fortuño & García-Izquierdo forthcoming) confirm this tendency, since some of the practising doctors who were interviewed admitted that they had lost their ability to be empathic with the passage of time. However, we agree with the increasing number of scholars and professionals who argue that empathic communication is a learned skill rather than only an innate predisposition (Marsden 2014; Ruiz-Moral et al. 2017), and that not only its acquisition should be fostered but also the ability to maintain it over time.

In the following sections, we will see how empathy can be shown both in oral and in written communication and will provide some strategies that can foster it. These will be useful for medical professionals, as well as for interpreters, translators and writers working in health care settings.

6.2 Empathy in oral communication

There is extensive literature that highlights the importance of empathy in oral communication skills in health care settings, from systematic reviews (Derksen et al. 2013) and focus groups with patients and health professionals (Derksen et al. 2018) to tests of health care practitioners' empathy through validated scales (Bernardo et al. 2018). Empathy in oral interactions has also been approached from translation studies, and more specifically, from the perspective of interpreting in medical and health care contexts.

Valero Garcés and Alcalde Peñalver (2021) conducted a systematic review of studies that relate empathy with the practice of interpreting in public services and concluded that real practice seems to contradict some aspects of the codes of conduct. Practice suggests including emotions when interpreting in patient–doctor encounters, while some codes of conduct advocate for neutrality. The authors affirm that professional conduct and empathic communication are not irreconcilable and that being able to deal with emotions is an added value that contributes to patients' understanding and satisfaction. Therefore, having an empathic attitude does not necessarily mean ignoring the codes of good practice. The authors add that empathy is even more relevant nowadays when the interpreting practice is increasingly being conducted remotely. (Valero Garcés and Alcalde Peñalver 2021).

It is important to be aware of the impact that managing distressed patients and emotionally complex situations can have on the professionals themselves, both physicians and interpreters (Wilkinson et al. 2017; Pérez Estevan 2022). A professional's excessive involvement with patients and their problems and a desire to help beyond their own means can have detrimental consequences. These can create exhaustion and burnout (Ruiz Mezcua 2014), and result in *compassion fatigue,* "being exhausted emotionally due to frequent difficult patient encounters, associated with the need for great attention and empathic

Suggestions for task. Exploring empathy in the medical consultation

In a medical consultation, have you ever experienced a situation (e.g. breaking bad news or dealing with a sensitive issue) in which empathy was particularly necessary on the part of the medical professional? What happened? How was empathy (or the lack of it) shown (non-verbal language, active listening, personal questions, etc.)?

listening" (Zenasni et al. 2012: 346). Empathy must involve the ability to distinguish the self from the other in order not to be misplaced in the patient's pain and emotions.

6.2.1 Strategies for building empathy in face-to-face interactions

As we have shown, empathy has been recognised as playing a key role in the training of health professionals in effective patient–doctor communication skills (Thompson et al. 2011, 2022; Brown et al. 2015; Tate & Frame 2019). One useful framework for this purpose is the Calgary–Cambridge Guide to interviewing patients (see Chapter 3); another is the CARE (Consultation and Relational Empathy) Measure (https://caremeasure.stir.ac.uk/), a patient questionnaire developed to measure health professionals' empathy in medical consultations.

In the next subsections, we include some strategies that help to foster empathy in face-to-face interactions, based on the literature review we have just discussed and the results of two GENTT research projects aimed at improving patient–doctor communication, both intra- and interlingually, in the context of three genres: fact sheets for patients, medical consultations and informed consent (Muñoz-Miquel 2019).

Listening actively and leaving room for questions

One of the most valuable strategies for showing genuine empathy is to listen attentively to the patient. This involves a series of verbal and non-verbal strategies that signal interest in the patient:

- Allowing patients to express how they feel, especially at the start of the consultation, instead of deliberately interrupting with closed questions, and leaving time for them to think before answering or to continue after pausing.
- Asking open-ended questions (e.g. the Kleinman questions; see Kleinmann et al. 1978). These do not limit the patient and give them a more active role. Explaining the rationale for these questions, when appropriate, can also stimulate unexpected responses.
- Facilitating the patient's comments by echoing or paraphrasing their last words.
- Leaving pauses; these help doctors to obtain more information and patients to perceive medical professionals as being more understanding.
- Maintaining eye contact – even despite physical barriers (e.g. a computer screen) – and listening actively, which is not compatible with reading or taking notes at the same time.

Providing reasoned explanations

It is important for health professionals to give the patient a road map of what will happen in a medical consultation; otherwise the patient may become anxious. A strategy for reducing anxiety is to state explicitly what is going to happen and always ask for permission. For example: *Now I'm going to explore your chest to see whether* [...] or *You may feel cold, but* [...].

Explanations and descriptions are also important when responding to patients' questions regarding their state of health. These should address patients' problems and avoid judging their behaviour. For example, when a patient asks about the reason for his knee pain, it is preferable to answer *I think you have some wear and tear, possibly a little early arthritis. So the best way to help reduce your pain is to lose weight*, rather than *You are overweight and that's why you have knee pain.* It is also important to provide appropriate justifications for medical instructions to ensure adherence to treatment and therapeutic processes. Patients are more likely to comply with instructions if they understand the reason for doing so.

Using plural pronouns and self-disclosure to establish trust and rapport

Using plural pronouns to indicate partnership is also a useful strategy for building rapport and showing empathy, for example when suggesting taking an action (*I hope you get better. Shall we meet in two weeks to see how you are getting on?*) or when describing symptoms (*That sharp pain we sometimes feel in our belly is due to gas*).

Sharing a bit about one's own experience when appropriate is also helpful as a way of showing that one really identifies with the patient's feelings and understands them while still being professional. This can be very useful when dealing with situations that are particularly stressful or shocking (when faced with an infertility diagnosis, for example: *I had infertility problems too and it really shook me up*).

Uncovering cues to emotional distress and eliciting concerns

When patients show emotional distress, a valuable response is legitimation and validation rather than ignoring it. *It's natural to feel fear at this point* is an example of a useful way of responding with empathy when patients overtly express their feelings. However, not all patients express their emotions, feelings, concerns and ideas directly. The health professional, therefore, needs to read behind their words and body language. A sigh, a shrug, a rueful smile or a different tone of voice may represent empathic opportunities, and it is necessary to respond to them with phrases that allow the patient to express their feelings (for example, *I noticed you sighed earlier on when I asked you about your uncle. Is that important to you?* or *And is there something that worries you about this pain?*). Echoing or repeating the end of their sentence when they pause can also be a good technique for encouraging further revelations.

It should be noted that it is important to show genuine empathy rather than just offering perfunctory responses that sound empathic without making any effort to clarify the source of the distress. To enhance empathy, it is also important to avoid expressions that imply that a patient's state, condition or situation is unimportant, trivialise what the patient is saying or expressing (*This is nothing; there are people who are much worse*) or indicate that one does not believe them (*It can't be that painful*). Otherwise, patients may feel that their concerns are being ignored and eliciting them can be an effective way of reducing their anxiety and emotional block.

Using a forecasting style when breaking bad news

Bad news, despite being stereotypically associated with a terminal diagnosis, can be of various kinds: a new chronic diagnosis, a worsening of a chronic illness, a need for surgery when pharmacological treatment is ineffective, to mention a few. Although there are some protocols for delivering bad news (such as the SPIKES[1] protocol or the ABCDE[2] mnemonic), this is an area in which less standardised communication strategies can be used, as preferences among patients vary greatly (Sparks et al. 2007; García-Izquierdo & Muñoz-Miquel 2015). Health professionals, therefore, need to be aware of their patients' patterns of information seeking or avoidance and to tailor the way they deliver information accordingly.

One strategy that proves useful is forecasting (Shaw et al. 2012), that is, being as descriptive, clear and honest as possible and avoiding abstract terms, euphemisms and complex medical terminology. This involves a staged delivery (providing some warning anticipations, such as *I'm afraid I have some difficult news*) to prepare the patient for what is coming but without delaying the news for too long; otherwise, patients may feel more anxiety and distress. Offering emotional support, allowing and respecting silence, giving space for questions and even using touch where appropriate can also be effective. Empathy in delivering bad news also means knowing how to strike a balance between reality and hope, even in the most serious medical scenarios. Hope does not necessarily refer to cure; in the context of serious diseases, it often refers to placing the disease within a time or discussing humane end-of-life conditions and dignified death.

Simplifying language and making explanations more understandable

In Chapters 4 and 5, we saw that asymmetries of knowledge are an important barrier affecting comprehension and rapport building. Some useful strategies to overcome this asymmetry are explaining or paraphrasing medical concepts (Montalt & González-Davies 2007), rephrasing in patients' modes of speaking or providing examples from everyday life for comparison and to enhance understanding. It is also helpful to use visual aids (such as drawings or pictures) to explain dosages or treatment plans and to check understanding by summarising patients' explanations or asking them to restate important pieces of information (e.g. by using teach-back and show-me; see Agency for Healthcare Research and Quality 2020).

Special care should also be taken with the words and expressions used with patients, given the devastating effect they can have on them. By way of example, a cancer patient who participated in the GENTT research projects explained that the first thing the surgeon said to her when they first met was *When are they giving you the poison?* (referring to chemotherapy), and this question, as she put it, "did her head in" (García-Izquierdo & Muñoz-Miquel 2015: 228).

Using non-verbal communication

The use of non-verbal language, as and when appropriate, is very helpful for giving an empathic response. Non-verbal language includes a wide range of elements, from posture, facial expression and eye behaviour to body movements, time allowed in turn taking and vocal cues. To enhance empathy, the following strategies prove effective: nodding to indicate understanding; smiling to show warmth; maintaining eye contact for active listening; touching or patting to show affinity, especially when breaking bad news; leaning forward to indicate attentiveness. Silence is also a valuable way of showing understanding and responding to emotions (Figure 6.1). Health professionals and interpreters can also take advantage of patients' non-verbal language to explore their feelings, ideas and concerns in greater detail. It should be borne in mind that cultural differences are especially evident in non-verbal language and that the communicative interaction patterns between health professionals and patients may differ even within the same language and culture.

- Listening actively and leaving room for questions.
- Providing reasoned explanations.
- Using plural pronouns and self-disclosure to establish trust and rapport.
- Uncovering cues to emotional distress and eliciting concerns.
- Using a forecasting style when breaking (bad) news.
- Simplifying language and making explanations more understandable.
- Using non-verbal communication.

FIGURE 6.1 Strategies for building empathy in oral communication.

Specific strategies for interpreters

In the field of interpreter training, frameworks have also been developed that provide strategies to meet the interpreter's needs in patient–doctor encounters. These needs can be classified into two main categories, according: the need for linguistic, cultural and communicative preparation; and the need for emotional preparation so as not to be personally affected by the patient's situation (Ruiz Mezcua 2014). In relation to the latter, empathy takes on a key role as a part of the interpersonal competence that has to be developed which involves: knowing how to listen to both the patient and the medical professional, dealing with empathy in situations of distress without this affecting the service provided, and developing skills to minimize the level of stress that interpreters may suffer (Valero Garcés & Alcalde Peñalver 2021).

The strategies shown in Figure 6.2 are used by professional interpreters to show empathy, as they contribute to building interpersonal relationships, promoting mutual patient–physician understanding and personalising communication. The strategies come from the contributions in the field of health care interpreting and mostly coincide with those to be developed by health professionals (Figure 6.1). Before moving on, we should consider that encouraging patients to express themselves in their mother tongue is the first and clearest sign of empathy that any professional in a health care setting can show. And in many cases, this can be achieved by hiring professional interpreters either in situ or remotely. As we saw in Chapter 4, not being understood and not understanding due to language barriers can be considered suffering related to care.

Interpreters also use other strategies in more particular contexts; for example, Gutiérrez et al. (2019) found that when doctors talked to Spanish-speaking parents and referred to the latter's children, interpreters used endearment to sound more familiar and show affection (e.g. when the clinicians used the child's name, interpreters used the terms *the baby girl* or *the little girl*). Parrilla Gómez and Postigo Pinazo (2018) also referred to using the patient's first name when addressing them even when the doctor does not do so. These are examples of strategies whose use will be clearly influenced by parameters such as the patient's culture, age, genre or ethnicity. Therefore, health professionals and interpreters should be aware of the different groups of patients they are addressing as well as the health care contexts and systems in which the interaction takes place, so as to avoid ethnocentrism (see Section 6.4 in this chapter).

Finally, we have to bear in mind that there are barriers that might affect communication and thus empathy. Researchers have reported on the negative effects on the development of empathic communication of the increasing

- Listening actively.
- Adding phrases that reiterate or clarify clinicians' statements (contextualisation).
- Adding reassuring or supportive phrases (encouragement).
- Simplifying language, making explanations more understandable and talking in a more friendly way.
- Asking if patients clearly understand the medical information they have received (checking understanding).
- Adapting clinicians' statements to be less direct and more polite (softening).
- Providing information in a gradual manner and using reflective pauses.
- Uncovering cues to emotional distress and eliciting concerns.
- Using forecasting when breaking bad news.

FIGURE 6.2 Strategies used by medical interpreters for showing empathy.
Source: adapted from Valero Garcés & Alcalde Peñalver (2021).

focus on effectiveness and productivity, as well as on technological advances (virtual consultations, increasing digitalization of medical procedures, etc.), rather than on the humane treatment of patients; other constraints on empathic communication during consultations include time pressures, heavy workloads, cynical views on the effectiveness of empathy and a lack of skill to show empathy (Derksen et al. 2013).

Suggestions for task. Showing empathy in fiction

Choose some scenes from the following TV series and film and reflect on the fictional use of the strategies for showing empathy.

- "House"
- "The Good Doctor"
- "New Amsterdam"
- *Patch Adams*

To what extent do you think these are authentic communication styles used in a real consultation? What can we learn from these characters?

6.3 Empathy in written communication

Although there is a growing consensus on the importance of written texts such as FSPs to supplement and even reinforce interactive verbal processes (Hirsh et al. 2009; García-Izquierdo & Muñoz-Miquel 2015), little attention has been paid to empathy in written communication, and research on this is scarce and seems to be in its early stages (see subsection 7.2.5 in Chapter 7). Empathy is more difficult to achieve in writing than orally because there is no room for conversational adaptation, that is, for perceiving emotions, identifying empathic opportunities (Du Pré & Foster 2015), and responding to them ad hoc (e.g. eliciting concerns, allowing questions, using non-verbal language).

Within translation studies, researchers have developed conceptual frameworks in which the receiver takes centre stage – intralingual or expert-lay translation (Zethsen 2018), user-centred translation (Suojanen et al. 2015), audience design (Mason 2000), patient-centred translation (Montalt 2017) – but they focus primarily on comprehensibility (see Chapter 5). Even though comprehensibility and empathy are very closely related – in fact, comprehensibility is the first and most evident sign of empathy – they are not entirely the same and may entail the use of different strategies to foster them. Although these scholars did not focus on empathy, some researchers have found in their studies that patients consider that fact sheets for patients are not written with them in mind (Hirsh et al. 2009; Fage-Butler 2015; Young et al. 2017) and would like more personalised genres that incorporate their experiences, knowledge and needs. From the perspective of the patient information leaflet, Herber et al. (2014) found that some patients perceived the risk and side effect language in the leaflets as frightening, and this provoked negative emotions that decreased their medication adherence.

These examples show that the way in which medical information is conveyed can significantly influence receivers' emotional response and understanding and thus their capacity to make well-informed decisions (Montalt & García-Izquierdo 2016). It is precisely in genres such as information leaflets and informed consent documents (see Chapter 2), which involve making a medical decision – taking a medication, undergoing a surgical procedure, participating in a clinical trial, etc. – that empathy is particularly relevant. When these genres are in the context of a highly sensitive medical specialty (e.g. oncology) or in key moments in the diagnosis or treatment of a patient (e.g. a life-threatening surgery), the need is even more crucial for information not only understandable but also empathic with the patient's feelings.

Other genres in which empathy is also very relevant are fact sheets for patients, which are often used to supplement the information provided orally by health professionals about a treatment or a disease. If these genres are not produced with the patient's needs and feelings in mind, translators and writers may introduce words or expressions which have no negative connotations for an average reader but which may sound alarming or even hurtful for a patient who is in a stressful and sensitive medical situation. One of the projects of the GENTT group referred to in Section 2.1 found that the fact sheets addressed to cancer patients that were written by nursing staff at the hospitals which participated in the study included words that the patients themselves considered "offensive", for instance *solvent* and *toxicity* in reference to chemotherapy treatments (García-Izquierdo & Montalt 2017: 606).

Empathy is also key in genres written by patients themselves and addressed to other patients, health professionals and the public: patient narratives. As we saw in Chapter 2, in these narratives, patients share their experiences in the course of an illness, a diagnosis or a treatment. These texts are characterised by conveying emotions and feelings, so empathy is very present. Patients' online forums and communities – in which patients share their medical experiences, as well as their opinions, views and feelings on a given disease or treatment – are another genre where empathy is truly evident, since patients seek not only useful health information in them but also empathetic support (Zhao et al. 2013). Through different linguistic, textual and iconographic strategies (such as metaphors, analogies or emoticons), patients show other patients that they put themselves in their shoes, view the situation through their eyes and truly understand them. Analysing these strategies can help us determine how to show empathy in written texts.

6.3.1 Strategies for addressing readers empathetically

Although some initiatives dealing with how to express empathy in the written mode can be found in fields such as business communication, only a few, as far as we are aware, focus on medical and health care settings. Fage-Butler and Jensen (2015) and Muñoz-Miquel et al. (2018) tackle the question of empathy, but they do not explore particular strategies in depth. For example, Fage-Butler and Jensen (2015) deal with patient and family-centred written communication in the palliative care setting and give recommendations on how end-of-life leaflets can reflect patients' and family caregivers' needs: that written materials be produced drawing on the skills of language, communication and document-design experts; that a lowest common denominator approach to texts, as the authors suggest, intended for a mass audience is applied to ensure that as many patients and family caregivers as possible can access the text; and that relevant medical terms be included but explained in the text.

The work by Lang and Esser (2012) is one of the few exceptions that focuses specifically on empathy in written texts addressed to patients. These authors argue that medical writers cannot merely impart facts but must also demonstrate that they comprehend the patient's emotions and rationale.

They suggest three principles of empathic texts: intelligibility, assuming the patient's perspective and credibility.

Intelligibility is the fundamental requirement of an empathic writing style because "failure to reach patients intellectually precludes engaging them emotionally" (Lang & Esser 2012: 305); this explains how comprehensibility and empathy are so closely related. Regarding the patient's position, this can only be accomplished "if the writer constantly reflects on how patients might perceive a concrete situation, that is, what the patient actually sees, hears, and feels" (Lang & Esser 2012: 306). Lang and Esser (2012) suggest that accessing patients' forums can help writers to gain insight into patients' needs. Finally, when talking about medical facts or research results, writers need to be credible, explaining concepts plainly yet precisely based on the latest medical knowledge and providing references. In this section, we include some strategies that help to address readers empathetically. These strategies come from a review of the above-mentioned studies, as well as from the results of the research projects of the GENTT Group referred to in subsection 6.2.1.

Adjusting tenor and personalising information

Using personal pronouns and making the subject of the sentence explicit to sound closer to the patient is sometimes preferred, especially in genres where patients are required to make an action or a decision, such as information leaflets or informed consent documents. It is also advisable in languages such as English and Spanish to use more active voice, especially when an action is required of the patient. For example, in a fact sheet about the side effects of a medication, *you can take paracetamol* would be better than *paracetamol is recommended.* In addition, abstract formulations should be replaced, when possible, with imagery (e.g. *keyhole technique* instead of *minimally invasive technique*).

Simplifying specialised terms and using plain language

As explained in Chapters 4 and 5, one of the most important asymmetries between patients and health professionals is that they do not share the same background knowledge. Health care professionals' extensive medical knowledge makes it sometimes difficult to communicate about their field in layperson's terms (Zethsen 2009). They therefore have to "struggle to distinguish between their own knowledge and that of the receiver" (Jensen & Zethsen 2012: 45).

According to patients, using specialised medical terms without providing an explanation makes them feel that their needs are not being taken into account, since no effort has been made to write in a language they can understand. Anticipating which terms and concepts will be difficult for them to understand and simplifying them therefore enhances not only comprehensibility but also empathy. De-terminologisation involves many potential strategies: synonymy, explanation, comparison, replacement by a more everyday term, etc. In the GENTT projects, patients usually preferred explanation or a more everyday equivalent but keeping the technical term in parentheses (e.g. *pins and needles (paraesthesia)*) because it allowed them to understand the concept while learning it. Finally, plainness is not at odds with veracity and precision, so, as stated before, facts, statements, results, etc., should be explained plainly yet precisely.

Avoiding ambiguous words

Ambiguous words are forms of expression that could be interpreted or defined differently by patients and health professionals, such as the word *rare* to describe a potential side effect of a medication. While a doctor may interpret rare as meaning, for example, a 5% chance of occurrence, a patient suffering significant emotional distress may think that the probability is higher, especially if their experience of illness is particularly negative. Therefore, written genres should be as explicit and clear as possible to avoid anxiety and misunderstanding.

Caring for lexical choices

As stated earlier, there are certain words or expressions with no impact for an average reader but which may sound alarming, hurtful or even offensive for a patient under a difficult medical situation. Written texts should opt for neutral lexical options when possible. The examples provided above about the terms *solvent* and *toxicity* can be quite illustrative. In a fact sheet for patients about the adverse effects of a drug, expressions such as *The main toxicity is neutropenia* could more empathetically say *the most common effect is a decrease in the number of white blood cells (neutropenia)*. Note also that this example simplifies the medical term but includes it in parentheses for patients' reference.

As writers, we should also take into account that even individual words not only convey information: they also awaken associations. A patient who suffers from migraines may describe them as being like *attacks* or *thunderstorms*. In such cases, generalising in a text about *pains* or even *complaints* would hardly demonstrate empathy.

Delivering content in small chunks and framing statements in a positive way

In order not to overwhelm patients with lots of information, texts – especially those which include a high degree of factual information like fact sheets or informed consent forms for clinical trials – should employ a single sentence to explain each important piece of information, thus transmitting the knowledge in small steps. According to the i-CONSENT Consortium, providing excessive information at once can amount to misinformation and hinder the communication process (Díez-Domingo et al. 2021).

When talking about facts, writers should consider that patients tend to respond better to statements when they are framed in terms of positive outcomes (Epstein & Street 2007). For that reason, preference should be given to statements framed in a positive way (e.g. *30% of patients will be free from this effect one year after treatment* may be more appropriate than *70% of patients will suffer this effect one year after treatment*) but always striking a balance between hope and reality, so as to avoid the information being perceived as unduly hopeful or pessimistic.

Adding information as needed

Including information that goes beyond mere instructions or descriptions of facts (even if this is not present in the original version) is useful. Like in oral communication, justifying medical recommendations in a way that avoids mere instruction and include examples to make certain complex or abstract concepts easier to understand contributes to empathy, fosters treatment adherence, encourages patients to take extra care when coping with side effects, etc. In addition, anticipating certain effects – especially when talking about medications – and their possible solutions may make patients feel more secure and more in control of the situation: it avoids premature anxiety and enables patients to be more involved in making informed decisions. Another communication strategy is to include sentences, or even whole sections if appropriate, in which the patient is urged to speak to the health care staff if necessary.

Providing sources for credibility when necessary

In the digital era, it is increasingly common for patients to search on the internet for health information, and even for self-diagnosis, with the risks this may incur. One of the reasons for these searches is often that patients do not have all their questions answered in the medical consultation or are not provided with written information to complement the explanations given orally by their doctors. In these cases, written texts such as fact sheets for patients, in addition to being ideal complements, can serve to provide reliable sources of information on the internet that patients can consult in case they need to expand their knowledge or resolve their doubts in relation to a specific aspect. This prevents patients from getting lost in the vastness of the web and finding information that is not suitable for them.

Using empowering metaphors and other rhetorical elements

In health care communication, metaphors are mainly used in two ways. First, to help make specialised concepts more comprehensible to lay people, and second, to express emotions and feelings. Metaphors can be very useful for describing symptoms and conveying specialised concepts. For example, when talking about migraines, expressions such as *thunderstorms in your head* would help to describe these pains. In patient narratives, metaphors help patients to capture their personal experiences of a disease. The following example illustrates this use: "How many people do we pass every single day who are *carrying around raging fires* – who have a passion or a pain inside that is so great they can barely contain it? For me, and for thousands of other people, *infertility is that raging fire*". Like other elements of medical language and terminology, metaphors are not always symmetrical across languages and cultures. Thus, medical writers and translators should be aware of these potential cultural variations when translating or writing medical and health care texts. In addition, foreign patients may find metaphors in another language hard to understand.

Euphemisms are another rhetorical element that can help to show empathy. Euphemisms are used to replace harsh or uncomfortable language with milder expressions or more pleasant-sounding words. Communicators can use them to convey sensitive information and talk about taboo subjects.

Including visual elements

Introducing visual elements, such as pictures, graphics, icons or illustrations can contribute not only to comprehension but also to empathy when they reassure patients. Even colours can be used to highlight habits that may be beneficial to the patient's health. In this regard, Saiz-Hontangas et al. (2016) and Prieto-Velasco and Montalt (2018) make interesting correlations between empathy and certain reassuring images in genres such as fact sheets for patients, which show the potential of images to play an important empathic role. An attractive layout with illustrations and graphical elements also mitigates the seriousness of some genres and make them more reader friendly. Providing information in formats other than written texts (webpage with hyperlinks, mobile app, videos, etc.) can also help to reach audiences which are keener to audio-visual and digital resources (e.g. children and teenager who participate in a clinical trial) (see Chapter 3).

Using fair and inclusive language

Medical writers and translators should use respectful language, especially when it comes to gender, race, ethnicity or sexual orientation. Thus, they should avoid unnecessary references to difference by using non-gendered alternatives unless those differences are key to the issue and avoid racial or ethnic stereotypes. Special attention should be paid to ableist language. Ableism is a negative bias against the physically challenged and differently abled, previously the disabled or handicapped. This negative bias leads to devaluation, discrimination and prejudice against people with physical, intellectual, or psychiatric disabilities (see Chapter 3).

Intentional or unintentional ableism is intertwined in our cultures, has different degrees and can take many different forms. Using ableist language when addressing patients, in particular ableist language that refers to them directly, is not fair and can have negative emotional impacts on them and hinder communication. Enhancing writers and translators' awareness of ableism can help them examine how it shows up in their own behaviour and communication processes, and explore ways to make positive, patient-centred changes. In response to ableism, *person-first language* (also called *people-first language*) puts the person before the disability and describes what a person has, not who a person is. It uses phrases such as *person with a disability, individuals with disabilities* and *children with disabilities,* as opposed to phrases that identify people based solely on their disability, such as *the disabled*; or *person with epilepsy* instead of *an epileptic.*

Another area of interest where empathy can be fostered is ageism. An example of ageism in language is the use of derogatory terms or stereotypes to describe older people. For example, using phrases such as *senile old man* can perpetuate negative stereotypes about ageing and contribute to ageist attitudes. Ageism can also be expressed in language through assumptions about older people's abilities or limitations, such as assuming that they are technologically incompetent or unable to adapt to new ideas. In addition, language that dismisses or belittles the experiences and perspectives of older people can reinforce ageist attitudes. Figure 6.3 summarises these strategies for translators and interpreters to build empathy in written texts.

- Adjusting tenor and personalising information.
- Simplifying specialised terms and using plain language.
- Avoiding ambiguous words.
- Caring for lexical choices.
- Delivering content in small chunks and framing statements in a positive way.
- Adding information as needed.
- Providing sources for credibility when necessary.
- Using empowering metaphors and other rhetorical elements.
- Including visual elements.
- Using fair and inclusive language.

FIGURE 6.3 Strategies that can help foster empathy in written texts.

TASK 6.1 SHOWING EMPATHY WHEN RESPONDING TO PATIENTS IN EMAIL CONSULTATIONS

Procedure

First, look at the enquiry that a patient has submitted to her doctor through email (see Materials below); then consider these questions:

- According to the parameters given in Section 6.3, do you think that the doctor's response has been empathic? Why or why not? Justify your answers.
- According to your experience, would a doctor in your own culture and language have responded in a similar way? Why or why not?

Materials

Dear Ms Bell,
Thank you for your email and questions. I am pleased to hear that John's breathing is better. And I appreciate that you told me that he hasn't been taking the inhalers regularly.

I recognize that it is difficult to accept that John has asthma. As we discussed last time when you both visited me there is no single test to confirm that someone has asthma. Diagnosis was made in his case based on symptoms characteristic for asthma (John was breathless for three months, was waking at night because of cough) and results of peak expiratory flow (blowing test) showing slight but significant narrowing of his airways.

I can't answer your question whether it would be good to stop the inhaler without seeing John and repeating the blowing test. Therefore, I suggest that you come to see me in the clinic in the next days (you can arrange it by email). We will then re-evaluate the diagnosis and discuss the use of inhalers.

In the mean time, you may find helpful reading the website about asthma in children http://www.besttreatments.co.uk/btuk/conditions/5838.html

Kind regards
Dr James Leeming

Please acknowledge reading this email and freely ask if anything is unclear.
*** Email is not appropriate for urgent advice – call Heaton surgery 0131 450 8702. ***
*** When the surgery is closed call NHS Direct 08 45 46 47. For emergency dial 999. ***

-----Original Message-----
From: Bell, Julie
Sent: Tuesday, 20 May 2004 05:01
To: Dr Leeming
Subject: John's breathing

Dear Dr Leeming
I still find it hard to believe that John has asthma. He is not breathless any more and I'm not sure whether this is actually due to the inhalers or it got better from itself. I am sorry to say but he hasn't been really taking very regularly the brown inhaler you prescribed, and the blue he used only a couple of times. This makes me wonder if he maybe anyway doesn't have asthma. I am writing to ask if he can stop taking the inhalers.
I look forward to your answer.
Kind regards
Julie Bell

Source: Car J, Sheikh A. Email consultations in health care: 2 – acceptability and safe application BMJ 2004; 329 :439 doi:10.1136/bmj.329.7463.439

As it happens with oral communication, there may be variations in the way empathy is shown in written texts depending on the language in which they are written or the culture they are addressed to. However, in oral interactions cultural differences are much more evident.

When patients understand the content of a given text and can identify with the language used in it, we can assume that the text fulfils its actual function: patients feel that their views are understood. Thus, they find it easier to comprehend and come to terms with their situation, understand and accept their condition, assess the advantages and disadvantages of different treatment options, engage in health-conscious behaviours, follow a therapeutic plan, etc.

In order to make texts really empathetic, it is essential to actively involve patients in the process of formulating, testing and improving texts addressed to or concerning them, since they are the ultimate health care recipients. In Chapter 7, we will explore the possibilities of research with patients to improve communication and make it more patient-centred.

6.4 Cultural variation in the expression of empathy

Culture is a crucial element in health care communication (see Chapter 1). Some of the communication aspects that may be affected by cultural differences are the amount of information embedded in the context, the content of the message, the way it is delivered and the paralinguistic features.

As a component of communication, empathy can also be influenced by culture. For example, in some cultures, it is a sign of empathy for doctors to make physical contact with patients when delivering bad news, while in others, the same attitude may be considered rude or even offensive. Emotional recognition can also vary across cultures. For example, although it is generally accepted that facial expressions of emotion communicate the same feelings, each culture may have different expectations about when, how, where and to whom facial expressions should be shown; for example, patients of Chinese origin tend to be uncomfortable being looked straight in the eye when talking to health professionals, due to a conflict avoidance principle. However, in some European countries, such as Italy or Spain, not looking a patient directly in the eye is perceived as a lack of interest on the part of the doctor.

Health care professionals, as well as medical writers, translators and interpreters, should be aware that empathy and the way it is expressed may vary from culture to culture. Therefore, they need to be careful when using oral and written strategies to manage emotions and show empathy, such as those we have been describing. This requires familiarity with the cultural background of the audience and the beliefs and practices of the health system in question. In this way, ethnocentrism – the use of one's own culture, ethnicity or nationality as a frame of reference for judging others – and stereotyping can be avoided, and empathic communication can be achieved.

TASK 6.2 ANALYSING EMPATHY IN WRITTEN TEXTS

Procedure

Analyse the following extracts, from a variety of sources, in which infertility is discussed. Identify what makes these texts more or less empathetic and why, taking into account the text genre to which they belong and the addressee.

Materials

Text 1

Infertility, the inability of a couple to conceive and reproduce. Infertility is defined as the failure to conceive after one year of regular intercourse without contraception or the inability of a woman to carry a pregnancy to a live birth. Infertility can affect either the male or the female and can result from a number of causes. About 1 in every 10 couples is infertile, or somewhere between 10 and 15 percent of the population.

Source: www.britannica.com/science/infertility

Text 2 What is infertility?

Infertility is when you have trouble getting pregnant or staying pregnant. Fertility problems can happen in women and men and can have many causes.

Infertility is common.

Some people have a hard time getting pregnant or staying pregnant. You're generally diagnosed with infertility if you don't get pregnant after 1 year or more of trying or if you have multiple miscarriages. There are treatments for many kinds of infertility, and many people go on to have a healthy pregnancy and a child.

Fertility isn't just a "woman's problem" or an issue with age. Lots of things can lead to infertility, and it can affect people of all sexes and ages. When a couple has a hard time getting pregnant, either person (or both people) is equally likely to be the cause. That's why both people are usually tested for infertility if a couple is having trouble getting pregnant.

Source: www.plannedparenthood.org/learn/pregnancy/infertility

Notes

1 The acronym SPIKES stands for Setting up, Perception, Invitation, Knowledge, Emotions with Empathy, and Strategy or Summary. See Rosenzweig (2012).

2 The ABCDE mnemonic stands for: Advance preparation, building a therapeutic relationship, Communicating well, Dealing with patient and family reactions, and Encouraging/validating emotions. See Vandekieft (2001).

Further reading

Fuller, M.; Kamans, E.; van Vuuren, M.; Wolfensberger, M.; de Jong, M. D. T. Conceptualizing Empathy Competence: A Professional Communication Perspective. *Journal of Business and Technical Communication*, 2021, *35* (3), 333–368. https://doi.org/10.1177/10506519211001125.

Jensen, M. N. Optimising Comprehensibility in Interlingual Translation. In *The Need for Intralingual Translation In Translation and Comprehensibility*; Maksymski, K.; Gutermuth, S.; Hanssen-Schrirra, S., Eds.; Frank & Timme: Berlin, 2015; pp. 163–194.

Kerasidou, A.; Bærøe, K.; Berger, Z.; Caruso Brown, A. E. The Need for Empathetic Healthcare Systems. *Journal of Medical Ethics*, 2021, *47*, e27. https://doi.org/10.1136/medethics-2019-105921.

Merlini, R.; Gatti, M. Empathy in Healthcare Interpreting: Going Beyond the Notion of Role. *The Interpreters' Newsletter*, 2015, *20*, 139–160.

Moudatsou, M.; Stavropoulou, A.; Philalithis, A.; Koukouli, S. The Role of Empathy in Health and Social Care Professionals. *Healthcare*, 2020, *8* (1), 26. https://doi.org/10.3390/healthcare8010026.

Sharma, A.; Lin, I. W.; Miner, A. S.; Atkins, D. C.; Althoff, T. Towards Facilitating Empathic Conversations in Online Mental Health Support: A Reinforcement Learning Approach. In *Proceedings of the Web Conference 2021 (WWW '21); Association for Computing Machinery*; New York, 2021; pp. 194–205. https://doi.org/10.1145/3442381.3450097.

Winter, R.; Leanage, N.; Roberts, N.; Norman, R. I.; Howick, J. Experiences of Empathy Training in Healthcare: A Systematic Review of Qualitative Studies. *Patient Education and Counseling*, 2022, *105* (10), 3017–3037.

7

STARTING RESEARCH IN PATIENT-CENTRED TRANSLATION AND COMMUNICATION

Overview of chapter

Throughout Chapters 1–6, we have identified a number of areas and aspects about which we have limited knowledge and where research is needed to make progress in improving patient-centred translation and communication. In addition to academic researchers, practitioners involved in research can contribute significant benefits to both academia and practice by bringing fresh real-world perspectives, experiences and challenges to scientific inquiry. We are addressing a diverse and multidisciplinary practical and academic audience, so the ideas in this chapter are aimed not only at translation and writing researchers and practitioners but also at those in health communication and health sciences more generally. This chapter is applicable to better understanding and improving clinical communication and patient–doctor interaction in both monolingual and multilingual settings, as well as to the training of health professionals, translators, interpreters and medical writers. We incorporate methods and tools from different areas of multilingual communication research and base the chapter on the idea that each of the research proposals presented can be adapted and applied to diverse cultural and situational contexts.

The first section offers brief presentations of selected research approaches, methods and tools that can be used to investigate patient-centred translation and communication (Section 7.1). Section 7.2 provides a schematic overview of some research areas of interest; for each of these areas, we present at least one research topic, some research questions and methods and some published research with the hope that they can guide readers in designing their own research. The chapter concludes with a section on resources for research

DOI: 10.4324/9780429299698-8

in patient-centred translation and communication that is not intended to be exhaustive but rather is aimed at providing the prospective researcher with information on websites, forums, databases and a bibliography on research methodology from which to build their own library of resources (Section 7.3).

7.1 Research approaches, methods and tools in patient-centred translation and communication

In this section, we provide an eclectic selection of research approaches (e.g. narrative analysis and critical discourse analysis), methods (e.g. interviews and surveys) and tools (e.g. readability formulas) that can be combined in multiple ways to form a specific study design to investigate relevant patient-centred translation and communication issues. Our aim is not to delve into the details of each of the approaches, methods and tools presented in any systematic way but to show the variety of options available to the prospective researcher. Therefore, we present them schematically, followed by suggestions of further reading for more detailed information on the theoretical background and practical applications of each of them.

7.1.1 Readability formulas

Readability formulas (see Chapter 5) are measures used to quantify the difficulty of texts: how easy or difficult they are to read and understand for the average reader in a given social group. They are widely used in journalism, research, health, law, insurance and industry. They originated with the US military, which developed its own set of formulas for technical training materials. Since then, many readability formulas have been developed in different languages and for different purposes, and thousands of studies on readability formulas have been published, demonstrating their strong theoretical and statistical validity.

Readability formulas statistically analyse several items: 1) the number of sentences in a given text; 2) the average sentence length per 100 periods; 3) the number of different words per sentence; 4) word length; 5) the number of sentences per paragraph and 6) vocabulary frequency lists. Ultimately, they compile those measures to determine a reading level for a given text: that is, at what typical literacy level can a reader read this text. Readers with more advanced reading skills can read and comprehend materials at higher literacy levels. One of the most commonly used formulas is the Flesch Reading Ease, developed in the 1940s by Rudolf Flesch (Jarret & Gaffney 2009).

Despite the success of readability formulas, they have always been at the centre of controversy. When the plain language movement in the 1960s led to legislation requiring plain language in public and commercial documents, a number of researchers attacked the use of readability formulas (Dubay

2004). From the point of view of patient communication research, readability formulas have limitations when used in isolation, as they focus exclusively on quantitative textual parameters and do not take into account the qualitative perceptions of individual patients. However, in a research study, these formulas can be the first step in establishing an average linguistic readability level of a given text and from there designing the study to validate (or not) this level of difficulty with qualitative data.

Further reading

DuBay, W. H. *The Classic Readability Studies*, 2007. https://eric.ed.gov/?id=ED506404.

DuBay, W. H. *The Principles of Readability*, 2004. www.researchgate.net/profile/William-Dubay-3/publication/228965813_The_Principles_of_Readability.

Jarrett, C.; Gaffney, G. *Forms that Work: Designing Web Forms for Usability*; Morgan Kaufmann, 2009.

Wang, L. W.; Miller, M. J.; Schmitt, M. R.; Wen, F. K. Assessing Readability Formula Differences with Written Health Information Materials: Application, Results, and Recommendations. *Research in Social and Administrative Pharmacy*, 2013, 9 (5), 503–516.

7.1.2 Corpus linguistics

A corpus is a collection of authentic texts selected and assembled for the study of language. Corpora are used to study regularities in at least three general areas: original and translated texts; translator and writer style; and regularities of languages and communicative situations, which is the most relevant in patient-centred translation and patient-centred communication. Corpus-based studies usually involve comparing at least two corpora. A basic distinction is made between parallel and comparable corpora. Parallel corpora are collections of texts in two or more languages that are translations of each other; each segment in one language corresponds to its equivalent translation in another language. Parallel corpora are primarily used for translation studies and machine translation research. Comparable corpora consist of texts in the same language or different languages that are not direct translations of each other. These corpora are compiled based on similar topics, genres, domains or time periods to enable comparative linguistic analysis.

Various tools are available for studying language and translation using corpora, such as concordances, clusters, collocates, frequency lists, keywords and n-grams. Software such as Sketch Engine or Wordsmith tools can be useful for this purpose. The GENTT research group at Universitat Jaume I built a corpus management tool specifically designed for specialised writers and translators (www.gentt.uji.es) based on the concept of text genre. The aim was to build a corpus with the largest possible number of text genres regardless of the number of words, which is the dominant criteria in many corpora. In corpus studies, quantitative methods often focus on the amount of data collected without taking into account the theoretical and descriptive contexts on which they should be based. This is why the GENTT group complements the research process with qualitative data.

Further reading

Bernardini, S.; Ferraresi, A. Corpus Linguistics. In *The Routledge Handbook of Translation and Methodology*; Routledge, 2022; pp. 207–222.
García-Izquierdo, I.; Borja Albi, A. A Multidisciplinary Approach to Specialized Writing and Translation Using a Genre Based Multilingual Corpus of Specialized Texts. *LSP & Professional Communication*, 2008, *8* (1), 39–64.
Zanettin, F. Corpora in Translation. In *Translation: A Multidisciplinary Approach*; House, J., Ed.; Palgrave, 2014; pp. 178–199.

7.1.3 Critical discourse analysis

Discourse is a broad term that refers to the way language (spoken, written and multimodal) is used in social interaction. There are different approaches to the study of discourse, but all are interested in how language is used to construct meaning, shape social identities and reproduce or challenge power relations. Critical discourse analysis (CDA) is a specific approach to the study of discourse that considers language as a social practice in a variety of settings, from everyday conversation and the media to politics and health care. Thus, CDA is not in itself a method but an umbrella term used to refer to a series of theories and practices that share certain principles in terms of their approach to the study of language. From the perspective of CDA and in contrast to corpus linguistics, texts are linguistic, not semiotic, units. This broader view of texts as semiotic units recognises that meaning is not solely derived from linguistic structures but also from the interplay of various signs and symbols. Texts can evoke emotions, convey cultural values and construct social identities through the use of semiotic elements beyond verbal language.

CDA is a powerful way for understanding how language is used to shape our perceptions and interpretations of the world. CDA aims to uncover the ideological assumptions and power relations embedded in language use. One of the crucial notions in CDA is ideology as a system of beliefs used to justify and maintain social order. Power is also a key concept and usually refers to the ability to influence or control the behaviour of others. Discourse analysts study how language is employed to support specific ideologies and how these ideologies can either justify or question established power structures. They also delve into how language is wielded as a means of exerting power, and how this power can either uphold or challenge social hierarchies.

Thus, one of the most fundamental premises of CDA is that language is not a neutral, abstract tool. Rather, it is a practice that is shaped by the social, cultural and ideological context. This means that the way we talk about health and illness is not simply a matter of personal preference, or professional practice, but is also influenced by the power relations and inequalities that exist in society. Language is used to represent the world in a particular way, and this representation can reflect and reinforce the interests of dominant groups in specific cultures and societies. In the context of health communication, this means that language can be used to promote certain health behaviours over others and to reinforce certain values and beliefs about health and illness. It can also mean that language is used to control or disempower patients and to reinforce asymmetries between patients and health professionals. CDA can be useful to unveil how language shapes social interactions.

Further reading

Bazzi, S. Critical Discourse Analysis. In *The Routledge Handbook of Translation and Methodology*; Zanettin, F.; Rundle, C. Eds.; Routledge, 2022; pp. 155–172.

Brookes, G.; Hunt, D., Eds. *Analysing Health Communication: Discourse Approaches*; Palgrave Macmillan, 2021.

Fairclough, N. *Critical Discourse Analysis*; Longman: London, 2013/1995.

Hatim, B.; Mason, I. *Discourse and the Translator*; Longman: London, 1990.

Van Dijk, T. A. Critical Discourse Analysis. In *The Handbook of Discourse Analysis*; Schiffrin, D.; Tanner, D.; Hamilton, H., Eds.; Blackwell: Oxford, 2015; pp. 466–485.

7.1.4 Narrative analysis

Humans are essentially storytellers, and all forms of communication are most usefully interpreted and evaluated from a narrative perspective (Fisher 1987, 1989). Narrative analysis is a research approach based on the premise that narrative meanings are inherent in human symbolic activities and are open to interpretation by research participants and investigators/observers (Yamasaki et al. 2014). This research approach focuses on the power of storytelling in shaping perceptions, attitudes and behaviours related to any field of human inquiry, including health and illness. As a research approach, it involves the systematic examination and interpretation of narratives or stories people tell about their health and illness experiences to understand the underlying meanings, structures and patterns within them. In narratives we typically find and can analyse plots, characters, motives, scenes, chronologies and values. Narratives can take various forms, including written or spoken texts, visual representations or combinations of media.

Riessman (2008) proposes four main analytic categories: thematic, structural, dialogic-performance and visual. Thematic analysis focuses on identifying the recurring themes or patterns that emerge from the narrative. These themes represent the central concerns, ideas or experiences conveyed through the narrative. Thematic analysis provides a way of categorising and organising the content of the narrative, allowing deeper insights into the narrator's experiences and the broader social or cultural context in which they are situated. Structural analysis examines the organisation and sequence of events within the narrative. It looks at the structure of the plot, the arrangement of events and how they contribute to the overall meaning of the story. Structural analysis identifies the turning points, climaxes and resolutions of the narrative and examines how these elements create a sense of coherence and convey the narrator's interpretation of events. Dialogic-performance analysis focuses on the interactive and performative aspects of narratives. It considers how narratives are constructed through a dynamic interplay between the narrator, the audience and the broader social context. Finally, visual analysis extends the scope of narrative analysis to incorporate non-verbal elements, such as photographs, videos and artwork. It examines how visual imagery is used to complement or extend the narrative's meaning.

Further reading

Charon, R. *Narrative Medicine: Honoring the Stories of Illness*; Oxford University Press: Oxford, 2008.

Charon, R.; DasGupta, S.; Hermann, N. *The Principles and Practice of Narrative Medicine*; Oxford University Press: Oxford, 2017.

Fisher, W. R. *Human Communication as Narration. Towards a Philosophy of Reason, Value, and Action*; University of South Carolina Press: Columbia, 1987.

Riessman, C. K. *Narrative methods for the Human Sciences*; Sage: London, 2008.

Yamasaki, J.; Sharf, B. F.; Harter, L. M. Narrative Inquiry. Attitude, Acts, Artifacts, and Analysis. In *Research Methods in Health Communication*; Whaley, B. B., Ed.; Routledge: New York; London, 2014; pp. 99–118.

7.1.5 Survey

A survey is a quantitative method used to obtain structured information directly from participants about the variables involved in research on a given population. The data obtained allow researchers to test relationships between variables (e.g. the effect of certain communicative attitudes of health professionals on patient health outcomes). Surveys require researchers to understand the topic well enough to know what questions to ask and what response options to offer. This basic level of understanding is best achieved through qualitative methods (interviews, focus groups, etc.), which can be helpful when designing a survey.

Surveys are often mistakenly used as a synonym for questionnaires, but they are not exactly the same: the survey is the task we want to do with a particular population (i.e. the study design), while the questionnaire is the main tool we use to do the task of surveying. The questionnaire consists of a list of questions, each with a range of answers, in a format that allows structured data to be collected from many participants. One of the main strengths of surveys is that they can provide a significant amount of quantitative data from large samples at a relatively low expense. This type of data allows statistical inferences and generalisations to be made about the whole population, but only if the sampling method used is appropriate and the sample is representative. However, there are some drawbacks to this method: although questionnaires can include open-ended questions to obtain qualitative information, they are not the best tools for obtaining explanatory data – opinions, personal experiences, etc.– unless they are followed up by other qualitative methods such as interviews.

Further reading

De Vaus, D. *Surveys in Social Research*; Routledge: London, 2013.
Morgan, S. E.; Carcioppolo, N. L. Surveys. In *Research Methods in Health Communication*; Whaley, B. B., Ed.; Routledge: New York; London, 2014.
Saldanha, G.; O'Brien, S. *Research Methodologies in Translation Studies*; St Jerome: Manchester, 2013.

7.1.6 Interview

Conversation is at the heart of this qualitative research method. Through conversation, we get to know other people and learn about their experiences, feelings, hopes and the world they live in. An interview is a planned conversation that has a structure and a purpose. Through interviews, researchers adopt a questioning and listening approach with the aim of gaining in-depth knowledge. Unlike other qualitative methods, interviews are one of the best tools for obtaining rich and multidimensional information (views, opinions, attitudes, perceptions, experiences) on a given topic from participants with different profiles.

One of the main strengths of interviews is that they allow the researcher to interact with participants to explore in depth the issues of most interest to their research and to make adjustments by observing how questions resonate with participants. Another strength of interviews is that they provide evocative and illustrative data from participants, so that direct quotations can be obtained that humanise the findings of a given study.

This method has some limitations. It is very time-consuming, not only for the researcher who has to conduct, transcribe and analyse the interviews, but also for the participants; indeed, recruiting valid participants is one of the major hurdles in this method. As a result, interview studies are often based on small numbers of participants who are often not representative samples, so results can rarely be generalised to wider populations. Another limitation is that interviews are self-reporting, which means that they provide insights into what participants say they believe or do, which may differ from what they actually think or do.

Further reading

Brinkmann, S.; Kvale, S. *Doing Interviews*, Vol. 2; Sage: London, 2018.
Donovan, E. E.; Miller, L. E.; Goldsmith, D. J. Interview/Focus Group. In *Research Methods in Health Communication*; Whaley, B. B., Ed.; Routledge: New York; London, 2014.
Kvale, S. *Interviews. An Introduction to Qualitative Research Interviewing*; Sage: London, 1996.
Saldanha, G.; O'Brien, S. *Research Methodologies in Translation Studies*; St Jerome: Manchester, 2013.

7.1.7 Focus group

Focus groups are a type of qualitative research in which a group of individuals who share a common characteristic such as the same illness are brought together to discuss a given topic. During focus groups, participants respond to the moderator's questions, engage in discussion among themselves and produce interaction data that can be useful to the researcher. Groups typically have between 6 and 10 participants, and sessions usually last around 1 to 2 hours.

Focus groups are very similar to collective interviews. What distinguishes them from interviews is that in focus groups the interactive nature of the activity and the synergies created among participants and the interviewer's role as a facilitator or moderator who gathers valuable information from the interaction among participants. Moderating focus groups requires careful preparation. Like interviews, focus groups can be more or less structured: when the discussion is structured, the moderator plays a more directive role, whereas when the discussion is more open, the moderator initiates topics but lets the interaction flow in the direction that the participants choose.

One of the advantages of focus groups is that the interaction among participants stimulates ideas and brings out diversity of opinions. This method is particularly useful for consolidating existing knowledge about participants' views, attitudes and beliefs; for finding out about why people think or feel the way they do and for brainstorming and generating new ideas. This is why focus groups are particularly useful in action research. However, this method has the drawbacks that the group leader – that is, the person who is the most knowledgeable or who has a more dominant attitude – may influence what is said or not said during the session, whereas more introverted participants may lose their voice, and that the results obtained during focus group sessions are not representative of the whole population, as is also the case with interviews.

Further reading

Donovan, E. E.; Miller, L. E.; Goldsmith, D. J. Interview/Focus Group. In *Research Methods in Health Communication*; Whaley, B. B., Ed.; Routledge: New York; London, 2014; pp. 21–41.

Flynn, R.; Albrecht, L.; Scott, S. D. Two Approaches to Focus Group Data Collection for Qualitative Health Research: Maximizing Resources and Data Quality. *International Journal of Qualitative Methods*, 2018, *17* (1), 1609406917750781.
Saldanha, G.; O'Brien, S. *Research Methodologies in Translation Studies*; St Jerome: Manchester, 2013.

7.1.8 Conversational analysis

Conversation analysis is a research method and theoretical approach in sociolinguistics and communication studies that involves the systematic study of naturally occurring spoken language in order to understand the structure, organisation and patterns of conversation (intonation features, pauses, etc.). Conversation analysis is concerned with the study of actual, real-life conversations and involves researchers collecting and analysing in detail the micro-level features of naturally occurring, pre-recorded conversations, for example the structure of individual turns, pauses, overlaps and other fine-grained aspects of conversational behaviour.

Conversation analysis emphasises the sequential organisation of talk, how one utterance leads to another in a real conversation such as a medical consultation. One of the central aspects of conversation analysis is the study of turn taking and how participants manage transitions between speakers. Repair is another crucial area of conversation analysis, that is, the processes by which participants deal with communication problems such as misunderstandings, errors and other disruptions in the flow of conversation.

Further reading

Antaki, C. Six Kinds of Applied Conversational Analysis. In *Applied Conversation Analysis. Intervention and Change in Institutional Talk*; Antaki, C., Ed.; Palgrave, 2011; pp. 1–14.
Couper-Kuhlen, E.; Selting, M. *Interactional Linguistics: Studying Language in Social Interaction*; Cambridge University Press: Cambridge, 2017.
Heritage, J.; Robinson, J. D. 'Some' Versus 'Any' Medical Issues: Encouraging Patients to Reveal Their Unmet Concerns. In *Applied Conversation Analysis: Intervention and Change in Institutional Talk*; Antaki, C., Ed.; Palgrave Macmillan: London, 2011; pp. 15–31.
Koenig, C. J.; Robinson, J. D. Conversation Analysis. Understanding the Structure of Health Talk. In *Research Methods in Health Communication*; Whaley, B. B., Ed.; Routledge: New York; London, 2014.

7.1.9 Dramaturgical analysis

The fact that we behave differently (play different roles) in front of different people (audiences) is a fundamental premise of dramaturgical analysis, a sociological perspective that originated in the work of Erving Goffman (1959), on which role play as an action-research method is based. This perspective views social interactions as performances on a stage, where individuals play their roles in a manner analogous to actors in a theatrical production. The central idea is that individuals engage in impression management, strategically presenting themselves to others in order to influence how they are perceived.

Key concepts in dramaturgical analysis include front and backstage, impression management, roles and scripts, audiences, props and setting, dramatic realisation and face-to-face interaction. Medical consultations can be seen as interaction rituals (in Goffman's terminology) in which the encounter is structured and patterned, often according to the doctor's clinical agenda. In the case of patient–doctor interactions in the consultation or hospital setting, roleplay (see subsection 3.1.1 in Chapter 3) is a useful way of exploring and understanding the asymmetries between the two roles and participants, and improving their performance.

In role plays, real-life patient–doctor interactions are devised, turned into scenarios and simulated in realistic ways. Through them, their participants (medical students, health professionals, interpreters, patients, etc.) can observe themselves as well as be observed by others who can provide useful feedback so that they can improve their communicative performance, either in the clinic or in educational contexts. As far as we are concerned in this book, role plays can be of two types: non-mediated (e.g. monolingual interactions where the participants share the same language) and mediated (e.g. bilingual or multilingual interactions where an interpreter is needed).

Role playing as an action-research method typically involves several stages. Firstly, scenarios are developed according to the educational and training needs in focus. Secondly, these scenarios are scripted or semi-scripted or simply left open to improvisation. Thirdly, they are performed, ideally with the help and participation of professional actors. While they are being performed, a process of external observation takes place. Fourthly, feedback is given by the observers and the actors involved in the simulations. Once the feedback has been discussed with all participants, the scenario is replayed as many times as necessary. This action-research method can provide practitioners and students (both in the medical and translation fields) with reflective and critical learning in a safe environment. Role playing can also be used to make patients aware of their assumed and ideal roles in their interactions with health professionals and interpreters.

Further reading

Goffman, E. *The Presentation of the Self in Everyday Life*; University of Edinburgh; Social Sciences Research Centre: Edinburgh, 1956.

Rønning, S. B.; Bjørkly, S. The Use of Clinical Role-Play and Reflection in Learning Therapeutic Communication Skills in Mental Health Education: An Integrative Review. *Advances in Medical Education and Practice*, 2019, *10*, 415–425.

Sapkaroski, D.; Mundy, M.; Dimmock, M. R. Immersive Virtual Reality Simulated Learning Environment Versus Role-Play for Empathic Clinical Communication Training. *Journal of Medical Radiation Sciences*, 2022, *69* (1), 56–65.

Skelton, J. *Role Play and Clinical Communication. Learning the Game*; Radcliffe Publishing, 2008.
Stokoe, E. Simulated Interaction and Communication Skills Training: The 'Conversation-Analytic Role-Play Method'. In *Applied Conversation Analysis: Intervention and Change in Institutional Talk*; Palgrave Macmillan: London, 2011; pp. 119–139.

7.1.10 Videoethnography

Videoethnography is a combination of videography (the practice of recording images with a video camera) and ethnography (a research method central to knowing the world from the standpoint of its social relations). Videoethnography has emerged as a valuable research method in patient-centred communication studies. It offers a unique lens for capturing and analysing the nuances of communication between health care professionals and patients in real-world settings. It provides a rich visual record of interactions, enabling researchers to observe nonverbal cues, body language and the overall dynamics of communication. Videoethnography captures interactions within their natural context, allowing researchers to understand how patient-centred communication unfolds in the complexities of health care settings.

Video-reflexive ethnography is a particular way of using videoethnograhy. The key distinction lies in their primary focus and objectives. Videoethnography is centred on the researcher's observation and understanding of social practices, while video-reflexive ethnography emphasises engaging participants in a reflective process using video as a tool for self-analysis and improvement. In Video-reflexive ethnography, participants view and discuss video recordings of their own actions, behaviours or interactions. This method aims to promote self-awareness, stimulate discussion and generate insights into the participants' own practices.

The four guiding principles underlying video-reflexive ethnography are *exnovation*, defined by Iedema et al. (2019: 12) as "the local ecology of care, that is, the accomplishment and complexity of everyday and taken-as-given care practices unfolding in the here and now"; *collaboration* as a participatory approach to data co-creation, analysis and redesign with stakeholders; *reflexivity* in the way of encouraging participants to re-view and re-imagine their practices and *care* in the sense of caring for participants' safety and crediting participants' contribution with relevance and significance. Its applications "range from improving clinical practices (such as handovers and infection control) in hospital wards to exploring what respect means in clinical consultations between patients and doctors, and what safety means for dying patients in palliative care contexts" (Iedema et al. 2019: 11).

Further reading

Grosjean, S.; Matte, F., Eds. *Organizational Video-Ethnography Revisited: Making Visible Material, Embodied and Sensory Practices*; Springer Nature, 2021.

Iedema, R.; Carroll, K.; Collier, A.; Hor, S. Y.; Mesman, J.; Wyer, M. *Video-Reflexive Ethnography in Health Research and Healthcare Improvement: Theory and Application*; CRC Press, 2019.
Liu, W.; Gerdtz, M.; Manias, E. Challenges and Opportunities of Undertaking a Video Ethnographic Study to Understand Medication Communication. *Journal of Clinical Nursing*, 2015, *24* (23–24), 3707–3715.
Woermann, N. Focusing Ethnography: Theory and Recommendations for Effectively Combining Video and Ethnographic Research. *Journal of Marketing Management*, 2015, *34* (5–6), 459–483.

7.2 Areas of interest

In this section, we explore seven areas of interest that we have chosen because they seem to be crucial for a better understanding and improvement of patient-centred translation and communication. The sequence that we have established in this section for each area is as follows: 1) area of interest; 2) possible topics to be investigated; 3) research questions (RQs) that derive from the topics and areas of interest presented and that can trigger specific research efforts, from a small study to a large project; 4) examples of methods that can be used to investigate some of the RQs proposed and 5) examples of published research that fully or partially address some of the topics or RQs presented. They are intended to provide hints on how to link topics, RQs and methods as well as literature reviews.

7.2.1 Patient-centredness

Patient-centredness is a crucial and evolving area of interest in health translation and communication research. As we argued in Chapter 1, patient-centredness emphasises a shift from a traditional biomedical model of health care to one that places the patient at the centre, considering their mother tongue, cultural background, preferences, values and involvement in decision-making. So important is this emerging area of interest that patients are even becoming proactive agents of medical research. The Patient-Led Research Collaborative, formed by patients experiencing long Covid-19, is a good example of this new role of patients engaged in conducting research. Emerging from the Body Politic Slack support group, they initiated the first long Covid study in April 2020. Members, experts in various fields including biomedical research, public policy and health activism, bring both professional knowledge and personal experience of Covid-19 to their work. Patient-generated research hypotheses are essential to patient-centred communication because they enable patients to be active participants in the research process. By allowing patients to contribute their perspectives, concerns and priorities, it ensures that research questions are relevant, meaningful and reflect patient needs.

Within patient-centredness, several topics need to be explored: for instance, the importance of the individual patient's mother tongue and culture in health care communication processes; the role of health literacy in patient health and well-being, particularly the relationship between patient-centred communication and clinical outcomes and the role of patients in decision-making about their health based on their ability to access and understand key information (see subsection 7.2.5). Another important unexplored topic is the expression of personal experiences of illness beyond the institutional context of the clinic. The measurement of patient-centredness in specific health care settings is yet another area where research can shed light and improve communication practices. Ethical issues related to key aspects of clinical translation and communication are also under-researched, for instance specific communicative situations and text genres such as informed consent (see subsection 7.2.4).

Examples of RQs

RQ1. What is the impact of patient-centred communication on patient well-being, recovery or adherence to treatment?

RQ2. To what extent can the level of health literacy of patients in a given health care system affect its efficiency?

RQ3. Do patients participate in shared decision-making processes that affect their health? How?

RQ4. What are the effects of using or not using the patient's mother tongue on patient understanding and satisfaction?

RQ5. Does the provision of translation and interpretation adequately cater to linguistic diversity in a given health care system?

RQ6. Is informed consent obtained in an ethical, patient-centred manner in specific clinical settings?

RQ7. Is the medical interview conducted in a patient-centred way, taking into account the patient's voice, concerns, values and preferences?

To investigate RQ5, employing focus groups and surveys among both patients and professionals within institutional settings offers a promising avenue. For RQ6, delving into videotaped scenarios alongside complementary focus group discussions can provide valuable insights into participants' perspectives and attitudes. Addressing RQ7 involves scrutinising medical consultations through videotaping, examining turn-taking dynamics via conversational analysis, and juxtaposing patient and doctor discourse through critical discourse analysis.

Some examples of published research

Altin, S. V.; Stock, S. The Impact of Health Literacy, Patient-Centered Communication and Shared Decision-Making on Patients' Satisfaction with Care Received in German Primary Care Practices. *BMC Health Services Research*, 2016, *16* (1), 1–10.
Crezee, I. H. M.; Roat, C. E. Bilingual Patient Navigator or Healthcare Interpreter: What's the Difference and Why Does It Matter? *Cogent Medicine*, 2019, *6* (1), 181087776.
Montalt, V. Ethical Considerations in the Translation of Health Genres in Crisis Communication. In *Translating Crises*; O'Brien, S.; Federici, F., Eds.; Bloomsbury Publishing: London, 2022; pp. 17–37.
Street Jr, R. L.; Makoul, G.; Arora, N. K.; Epstein, R. M. How Does Communication Heal? Pathways Linking Clinician-Patient Communication to Health Outcomes. *Patient Education and Counseling*, 2009, *74* (3), 295–301.

7.2.2 Culture and context

As we showed in Chapter 1, context is crucial in all studies concerned with the analysis of communication, and the field of patient communication is no exception. As the proponents of systemic functional linguistics have pointed out (Halliday & Hasan 1985; Halliday & Matthiessen 2013), in order to understand communicative exchanges properly, it is necessary to understand the contexts in which they take place, which these authors divide into two large dimensions: the broader cultural context and the context of the specific situation. In this area, some issues and research questions arise that may be relevant for determining to what extent an adequate knowledge of the context is key to ensure the success of the communication.

Among the research topics, we can highlight the influence of cultural beliefs on patient–doctor communication, the perceptions of patients from a given culture on the functioning of the health system or how health legislation can regulate communication.

Examples of RQs

RQ1. What are the patients' dominant values and beliefs about health care in areas such as reproductive health, abortion, mental health and other sensitive issues in a given culture?
RQ2. How do patients' rights and duties, as defined in regulatory frameworks, determine the functioning of communication in specific health systems?
RQ3. What are the dominant roles and attitudes of professionals and patients in a given health system? What are the asymmetries between them?
RQ4. What are the degrees of explicitness in the delivery of health information addressed to patients and to what extent the context plays a crucial role in making sense of it in different health cultures?

RQ5. How are stereotypes, taboos and stigma regarding health and illness reflected in language and communication?
RQ6. How is non-verbal communication during consultations (e.g. physical distance, eye contact) used by patients and professionals from different cultures?

To address RQ1, we propose analysing a corpus of texts aimed at patients on sexuality among young people with cancer; contrasting the findings with insights from a focus group of people in similar circumstances could enrich our understanding. RQ2 would benefit from a descriptive analysis of relevant legislation on patient information, complemented by a survey assessing both professionals' and patients' awareness of and compliance with their respective rights and responsibilities. RQ3 could be explored using qualitative methods such as interviews or surveys involving both professionals and patients. This approach aims to elucidate professionals' perceptions of their own communication roles and patients' perspectives on this. In addressing RQ5 through CDA, analysts could explore potential discrimination faced by specific groups of patients or citizens, taking into account factors such as culture, language proficiency, gender, socioeconomic status and functional diversity.

Some examples of published research

Domaradzki, J. Patient Rights, Risk, and Responsibilities in the Genetic Era – A Right to Know, a Right Not to Know, or a Duty to Know? *Annals of Agricultural and Environmental Medicine*, 2015, *22* (1).
Giordano, M. Healthcare Power of Attorney and the Living Will: Comparing and Contrasting Medical-Legal Genres. In *Professional Discourse Across Medicine, Law, and Other Disciplines: Issues and Perspectives*; Girolamo Tessuto, R. A.; Bhatia, V. K., Eds.; Cambridge Scholars Publishers, 2023; p. 110.
Kapoor, A.; McKinnon, M. The Elephant in the Room: Tackling Taboos in Women's Healthcare. *Journal of Science Communication*, 2021, *20* (1), C10.
Traumer, L.; Jacobsen, M. H.; Laursen, B. S. Patients' Experiences of Sexuality as a Taboo Subject in the Danish Healthcare System: A Qualitative Interview Study. *Scandinavian Journal of Caring Sciences*, 2019, *33* (1), 57–66.

7.2.3 Education and training

One of the main conclusions drawn from the different chapters in this book is that a lack of communicative and cultural competence on the part of health professionals negatively influences the way they communicate – both orally and in written – with patients. This can lead to a lack of patient-centredness, poor patient satisfaction and adherence to treatment, increased anxiety and suffering and other undesirable effects on patients' health. For this reason, the acquisition of communication skills through formal training is essential to promote patient-centredness and, in turn, better health outcomes.

Some of the topics that need to be further explored through research are education and training in communication skills and methods, not only for health professionals but also for translators, interpreters and medical writers. Cultivating cultural competence through education and training programmes is another important area that needs to be explored in greater depth. These efforts are critical to improving the quality of health care and ensuring effective communication with diverse patient populations.

Examples of RQs

RQ1. To what extent do education and training in communicative and cultural competence improve health outcomes in patients?
RQ2. How can communicative and cultural competence be taught and acquired?
RQ3. Does the university curriculum address the acquisition of communicative and cultural competence by health students? How and to what extent?
RQ4. Do health professionals have and use effective communication skills in their interactions with patients during consultations? If not, do they receive continuous counselling and training in their workplaces?
RQ5. Do health professionals perceive the importance of being sensitive to different languages and cultures during consultations? What do they think about the use of the patient's mother tongue?
RQ6. What do patients think about the communication skills of their health professionals?

RQ2 could be investigated using role play: students of medicine and other health-related degrees could take part in simulations of medical consultations with professional actors playing different patient roles. These role plays could then be analysed by communication experts who would provide students with useful feedback for helping them to improve their communication skills through repeated performances of the same simulated consultations. In addition to role plays, narrative analysis of patients' narratives can be used to make health professionals aware of patients' personal experiences of illness. To respond to RQ3, the researcher could first collect and analyse a corpus of syllabi of the university medical degrees offered in a given country or region to identify which communicative, ethical and cultural competences (if any) students are expected to acquire. RQ4 can be explored using video-reflexive ethnography; in addition, conversational analysis can be performed to describe aspects such as turn taking, politeness or repairing strategies, to mention just a few. RQ5 can be explored by means of focus groups and in-depth interviews to analyse if health professionals consider that being sensitive to different languages and cultures during consultations is important and why.

Some examples of published research

Crezee, I. Semi-Authentic Practices for Student Health Interpreters. *Translation & Interpreting*, 2015, *7* (3), 50–62.

Crezee, I.; Jülich, S. Exploring Role Expectations of Healthcare Interpreters in New Zealand. In *Interpreting in Legal and Healthcare Settings: Perspectives on Research and Training*; John Benjamins, 2020; pp. 211–241.

Deveugele, M. Communication Training: Skills and Beyond. *Patient Education and Counseling*, 2015, *98* (10), 1287–1291.

García-Izquierdo, I.; Montalt, V. Cultural Competence and the Role of the Patient's Mother Tongue: An Exploratory Study of Health Professionals' Perceptions. *Societies*, 2022, *12*, 53. *Cultural Competence in Healthcare and Healthcare Education, 89.*

Kreps, G. L. Communication and Health Education. In *Communication and Health. Systems and Applications*; Ray, E. B.; Donohew, L., Eds.; Routledge, 2013; pp. 187–203.

7.2.4 Genres

In Chapter 2, we discussed the centrality that we believe the concept of text genre has as a conceptual tool that allows us to address all aspects of understanding how communication works. Genre, as a multifaceted concept that combines formal (linguistic-textual), communicative (senders and receivers) and cognitive (content and ideology) considerations, can help us to comprehensively characterise the pragmatic intentionality of those who participate in patient-centred communication.

There are many compelling avenues of research in this area. Firstly, exploring the intricacies of health discourse across genres and genre systems within specific cultural milieus is promising. Secondly, exploring the linguistic subtleties, writing conventions and norms that shape genres in different languages is a fascinating area ripe for exploration. Finally, examining the influence of emerging genres on the dynamics PPC offers an intriguing dimension for further exploration.

Examples of RQs

RQ1. What are the genres operating in a given health care system?
RQ2. What are the genre systems that configure communication in given processes or procedures?

RQ3. To what extent is the delivery of specialised knowledge to the lay public facilitated through specific genres in different languages and cultures?
RQ4. How can emerging genres addressed to patients contribute to giving voice to them and to improving communication?
RQ5. What are the perceptions of participants (health professionals and patients) in given genres, such as the informed consent and the consultation, about the way communication is carried out?
RQ6. How do various genres addressed to patients differ regarding the amount of medical terminology they typically contain?
RQ7. Which are the most typical phraseological expressions in given genres?

RQ1 and RQ2 could be addressed using a number of research methods. Firstly, we could manually map the genres relevant to our investigation; we could also analyse a corpus of relevant genres within a particular health care system or, in the case of RQ2, within public health campaigns or medical procedures such as surgical interventions. This analysis could span multiple languages, using comparable corpora to explore cultural variation in different contexts.

In addition, we could explore RQ2 using CDA to examine how public health campaigns frame issues such as smoking and the subsequent impact on attitudes and behaviours. CDA researchers can examine how the media frame health risks and their influence on public risk perceptions. They can also examine the portrayal of illness in health communication and its impact on individuals' experiences of illness. For example, mental illnesses are often portrayed in the media as stigmatised and shameful, whereas diseases such as cancer are portrayed as heroic and inspiring. It is important to recognise that these dynamics often differ across languages and cultures.

In response to RQ3, CDA provides a valuable method for examining how genres portray patients as either experts or laypeople. Similarly, RQ7 can be explored using narrative analysis, which examines the organisation of characters and plots in temporal and spatial dimensions. This approach allows us to explore various elements, including the presence of archetypal characters such as heroes and antagonists, the setting of the narrative, the logic behind the sequence of events, the motivations of the narrators, the underlying worldviews, the cultural nuances embedded in the narratives and the therapeutic aspects of storytelling.

Some examples of published research

Best, M.; Jenkins, E. The Value of Involving Patients and the Public in Writing Patient Information. *Pharmaceutical Journal*, 2016, *297* (7898), 1–4.

Borja, A.; García-Izquierdo, I.; Montalt, V. Research Methodology in Specialized Genres for Translation Purposes. *The Interpreter and Translator Trainer*, 2009, *3* (1), 57–77.

Bos, L.; Marsh, A.; Carroll, D. Co-Design of Patient Information Leaflets (PILs): A Qualitative Exploration of Patient and Public Involvement (PPI) in PIL Development. *Health Expectations*, 2019, *22* (5), 1075–1082.
García-Izquierdo, I.; Bellés-Fortuño, B. Improving Clinical Communication: A Qualitative Study on the Informed Consent. *RLYLA*, 2024, 19, 71-83.
García-Izquierdo. I.; Borja, A. La comunicación en contextos de salud: generación de recursos tecnológicos multilingües para la mejora de la eficacia comunicativa del Consentimiento Informado. Cadernos de Tradução, 2024, 44, e95247.
García-Izquierdo, I. Metadiscourse in Informed Consent: Reflections for Improving Writing and Translation. *GEMA Online Journal of Language Studies*, 2022, *22* (4), 161.
García-Izquierdo, I.; Montalt, V. Understanding and Enhancing Comprehensibility in Texts for Patients in an Institutional Health Care Context in Spain: A Mixed Methods Analysis. *RESLA. Revista Española de Lingüística Aplicada/Spanish Journal of Applied Linguistics*, 2017, *30* (2), 592–610.
Spinuzzi, C. Describing Assemblages: Genre Sets, Systems, Repertoires, and Ecologies. *Computer Writing and Research Lab*, 2004, White Paper Series: #040505–2, 1–9.

7.2.5 Comprehensibility and emotions

Chapters 5 and 6 showed that the ways in which medical information is conveyed can significantly influence receivers' understanding and their emotional response: the messages is that when communicating with patients and translating/writing for them, special attention must be paid to comprehensibility and emotions. The information provided – either orally or written– has to be formulated in such a way that a lay audience (patients, family members, the general public, etc.) can understand it but also feel reassured, respected and treated in a humane way. To achieve this, translators, writers and health professionals have to identify the needs of the target audience and determine which means – grammatical, terminological, stylistic, textual, pragmatic, non-verbal – will make communication more comprehensible, empathetic and attractive.

Some of the topics that need to be further explored through research are the following: empathy and affective aspects of genres for or involving patients, comprehension of medical information, the strategies that make oral and written communication comprehensible and empathetic, the influence of culture on the understanding of specialised knowledge or the use of empathy by health professionals, among others.

Examples of RQs

RQ1. Are genres addressed to patients really comprehensible and empathetic to them?
RQ2. What strategies (both verbal and non-verbal) are used in communication that is considered understandable and empathetic?

RQ3. What do patients and health professionals think about the value of empathy in clinical communication?
RQ4. Do health professionals use understandable and empathetic language in their interactions with patients?
RQ5. How do patients themselves show empathy, both verbally and non-verbally?
RQ6. How does culture influence the way empathy is shown and understood?

To address RQ1 regarding the level of comprehensibility, we can choose to select a corpus of texts aimed at patients and apply readability formulas. In addition, qualitative analysis can be applied, using focus groups in which patients provide feedback on the readability and usability of the text. RQ4 involves the use of validated scales and questionnaires to measure the level of empathy in medical consultations, coupled with interviews with both patients and health care professionals. To investigate RQ5, a corpus of patient interactions from online forums dedicated to a specific disease and conversation analysis can provide insights into how empathy is expressed among patients.

Some examples of published research

Fitchett, G.; Emanuel, L.; Handzo, G.; Boyken, L.; Wilkie, D. Care of the Human Spirit and the Role of Dignity Therapy: A Systematic Review of Dignity Therapy Research. *BMC Palliative Care*, 2016, *15* (1), 1–11.

García-Izquierdo, I.; Montalt, V. Understanding and Enhancing Comprehensibility in Texts for Patients in an Institutional Health Care Context in Spain: A Mixed Methods Analysis. *Revista Española de Lingüística Aplicada/Spanish Journal of Applied Linguistics*, 2017, *30* (2), 592–610.

Nordtug, M.; Møller, J. E.; Matthiesen, S. S.; Brøgger, M. N. Oralizations in E-Mail Consultations: A Study of General Practitioners' Use of Non-Verbal Cues in Written Doctor-Patient Communication. *Catalan Journal of Communication & Cultural Studies*, 2021, *13* (2), 195.

Tercedor Sánchez, M.; Láinez Ramos-Bossini, A. Resemblance Metaphors and Embodiment as Iconic Markers in Medical Understanding and Communication by Non-Experts. In *Operationalizing Iconicity. Iconicity in Language and Literature, 17*; Perniss, P.; Ljungberg, C., Eds.; John Benjamins, 2020; pp. 265–289.

7.2.6 Audience analysis

As we have seen in Chapter 4, one of the key aspects for a proper understanding of health communication is to consider the diverse configurations of audiences. Each patient is unique according to age, gender, ethnicity or national culture, literacy level and professional culture or illness, among many other variables. It is therefore very important that we know how to distinguish the characteristics of the audiences of certain genres (written or oral) when writing or translating them.

Among the research topics that we can highlight in this area are the configuration of the audience in a specific health culture and its characterisation, the existence of specific communication needs for certain groups of patients or the analysis of specific problematic aspects that can make communication difficult.

Examples of RQs

RQ1. In a given health care system, are there communication policies that encourage addressing specific groups of patients in an adequate way?
RQ2. Which are the dominant criteria when deciding how to group patients with different circumstances in order to address them adequately?
RQ3. What is the level of health literacy of the population in a given health care system?
RQ4. Which expectations, purposes and needs do specific audiences have regarding communication?
RQ5. How are specific audiences (children, chronic patients, patients with disabilities, etc.) addressed in given communicative situations?
RQ6. How do we address a diverse audience in public health communication where everybody must be included?
RQ7. What is the level of satisfaction of users of health services with the way they are addressed?

To address RQ4, we can conduct audience analysis by exploring the expectations and information needs of patients with the same condition, such as stomach cancer. Qualitative research methods such as focus groups can facilitate this exploration. In addition, we can use critical discourse analysis to explore the underlying factors that shape these expectations, such as age, literacy levels and cultural taboos associated with the disease. For RQ7, we could use focus groups and surveys tailored to patients receiving specific health services or experiencing specific health conditions.

Some examples of published research

Al Shamsi, H.; Almutairi, A. G.; Al Mashrafi, S.; Al Kalbani, T. Implications of Language Barriers for Healthcare: A Systematic Review. *Oman Medical Journal*, 2020, *35* (2), e122.

García-Izquierdo, I.; Montalt, V. Cultural Competence and the Role of the Patient's Mother Tongue: An Exploratory Study of Health Professionals' Perceptions. *Societies*, 2022, *12* (2), 53.
Kim, J. E.; Lee, Y. M.; Park, K. H. The Impact of Patient-Centered Communication on Patient Satisfaction and Health Literacy: A Systematic Review and Meta-Analysis. *International Journal of Environmental Research and Public Health*, 2019, *16* (10), 1808.
Mohan, A.; Riley, M. B.; Boyington, D.; Johnston, P.; Trochez, K.; Jennings, C.; Kripalani, S. Development of a Patient-Centered Bilingual Prescription Drug Label. *Journal of Health Communication*, 2013, *18* (sup 1), 49–61.
Selman, L. E.; Brighton, L. J.; Sinclair, S.; Karvinen, I.; Etkind, S. N.; Bristowe, K.; Murtagh, F. E. Patients' and Caregivers' Needs, Experiences, Preferences and Research Priorities in Spiritual Care: A Focus Group Study Across Nine Countries. *BMC Palliative Care*, 2019, *18* (1), 1–15.
Street Jr, R. L.; Gordon, H. S.; Ward, M. M.; Krupat, E.; Kravitz, R. L. Patient Participation in Medical Consultations: Why Some Patients Are More Involved Than Others. *Medical Care*, 2005, *43* (10), 960–969.

7.2.7 Multimodality and accessibility

In Chapter 3, we approached multimodal texts and communicative events as composed of multiple semiotic resource such as still and moving images, speech, writing, layout, gesture and proxemics. Web pages, for example, may contain linguistic elements, images, colour, layout, animation, voice or music, each of which is a 'mode'.

As technology continues to evolve, multimodality in health communication will play an increasingly important role in improving patient-centred care and health outcomes. Researchers are exploring the use of virtual reality, augmented reality and artificial intelligence to create immersive and engaging communication experiences for patients. In addition, research is focused on developing personalised communication strategies based on individual patient preferences and needs.

Integrating multimodal communication into patient-centred care can lead to improved patient outcomes, increased satisfaction and greater equity in health care. By harnessing the power of multiple communication channels, health care providers can build stronger relationships with patients, promote informed decision-making and foster more collaborative approaches to health care. One of the main themes of multimodal research in translation studies is accessibility (O'Sullivan 2013), which is highly relevant in patient-centred communication and translation, where it is seen not only as a challenge but also as a very productive resource.

One of the most relevant topics is the fact that multimodality can meet the needs of diverse patient groups and ensure inclusivity. A second topic is the benefits that multimodality can bring to patients' understanding of medical information and satisfaction with health care. Another topic of interest is the emergence of new multimodal genres and the transformation of the existing ones due to technological developments. Finally, translators, interpreters and medical writers are faced with the challenge of having to combine multiple modes to address target audiences and make decisions where there may be substantial changes between source and target modes.

Examples of RQs

RQ1. How can multimodal solutions improve patients' understanding of medical information and increase their satisfaction with care?
RQ2. Do health professionals make use of multimodal resources in their interactions with patients in clinical contexts?
RQ3. How can multimodal approaches bridge cultural and linguistic barriers to ensure equitable access to quality health care for all patients?
RQ4. How can images and diagrams complement verbal communication to make it more inclusive for diverse groups of patients (e.g. patients with hearing impairments)?
RQ5. Do patients feel more involved and empowered when they can access information and make decisions through different communication channels and modes?
RQ6. How do specific genres become multimodal through the development of technological innovations (e.g. electronic informed consent)?
RQ7. How do translators and interpreters perceive the need for multimodal (intersemiotic) translation?

RQ1 can be investigated through role plays in which simulated patients explore their understanding of medical information by means of different modes, channels, media, etc. To respond to RQ6, multimodal corpus analysis can be useful for describing both inter- and intralingual communication processes and how different modes and media complement each other and carry out different functions. To respond to RQ7, in-depth interviews and focus groups can shed light on how translators and interpreters deal with multimodal translation and address the specific needs of target audiences in real contexts.

Some examples of published research

Boivin, A. C. N.; Cohen Miller, A. Inclusion and Equity with Multimodality During Covid-19. In *Keep Calm, Teach On: Education Responding to a Pandemic*; Vyortkina, D.; Collins, N.; Reagan, T., Eds.; Information Age Publishing, 2022; p. 89.

Cluley, V.; Bateman, N.; Radnor, Z. The Use of Visual Images to Convey Complex Messages in Health Settings: Stakeholder Perspectives. *International Journal of Healthcare Management*, 2021, *14* (4), 1098–1106.
Montalt, V.; García-Izquierdo, I. Exploring the Links between the Oral and the Written in Patient-Doctor Communication. In *Medical Discourse in Professional, Academic and Popular Settings*; Ordóñez, P.; Edo-Marzá, N., Eds.; Multilingual Matters, 2016; pp. 103–125.
O'Sullivan, C. Introduction: Multimodality as challenge and Resource for Translation. *The Journal of Specialised Translation*, 2013, *20*, 2–14.
Yadav, S. P.; Yadav, S. Image Fusion Using Hybrid Methods in Multimodality Medical Images. *Medical & Biological Engineering & Computing*, 2020, *58*, 669–687.

7.2.8 A final note on machine translation and artificial intelligence

Another area of significant interest is the field of machine translation and artificial intelligence (AI) in health care. Chatbots such as Google's Bards GPT are increasingly being used by both patients and health care professionals. These AI-powered tools offer innovative solutions for health care communication and information dissemination. By leveraging machine translation, they enable seamless interactions between individuals and health care systems, facilitating the exchange of vital health-related information and support. However, it's important to recognise the risks and challenges associated with AI in patient-centred communication and translation. Concerns such as data breaches, translation inaccuracies and the potential for misinterpretation of medical information highlight the need for careful implementation and ongoing evaluation of AI-driven solutions. As technology continues to advance, the integration of AI-driven solutions such as chatbots holds great promise for improving the accessibility, efficiency and effectiveness of health care communication but must be approached with caution to mitigate potential risks and challenges.

Research questions in this emerging field cover various aspects, such as understanding health care professionals' perceptions of the effectiveness and reliability of AI and machine translation tools in facilitating patient-centred communication. In addition, researchers seek to identify the main challenges and barriers associated with implementing these technologies in patient-centred translation and communication. Exploring patients' perspectives on the use of AI and machine translation in accessing health care information and communicating with health care providers is another important area of research. Researchers may also seek to identify effective strategies to ensure that AI and machine translation tools adequately support patient-centred communication while maintaining accuracy and cultural sensitivity. Finally, research can examine the impacts of integrating AI and machine translation on the role of language experts and interpreters in patient-centred translation and communication.

Some examples of published research

Haddow, B.; Birch, A.; Heafield, K. Machine Translation in Healthcare. In *The Routledge Handbook of Translation and Health*; Routledge, 2021; pp. 108–129.
Khoong, E. C.; Rodriguez, J. A. A Research Agenda for Using Machine Translation in Clinical Medicine. *Journal of General Internal Medicine*, 2022, *37* (5), 1275–1277.
Pym, A.; Ayvazyan, N.; Prioleau, J. Should Raw Machine Translation Be Used for Public-Health Information? Suggestions for a Multilingual Communication Policy in Catalonia. In *Language Policies for Social Justice*; Mellinger, C. D.; Monzó-Nebot, E., Eds.; Special Issue. *Journal of Language Rights & Minorities, Revista de Drets Lingüístics I Minories*, 2022, *1* (1–2): 71–99.
Zappatore, M.; Ruggieri, G. Adopting Machine Translation in the Healthcare Sector: A Methodological Multi-Criteria Review. *Computer Speech & Language*, 2023, 101582.

7.3 Some resources for research in patient-centred translation and communication

In this final section, we provide a brief selection of materials and resources that can help the budding researcher take the first steps on their research journey.

7.3.1 Basic references

You can get a general idea of what academic research involves in practice by reading Booth, W. C., Colomb, G. G., & Williams, J. M. (2008). *The craft of research*. University of Chicago Press. You can then delve into more detailed methodological and thematic accounts in the following handbooks and manuals:

Alves, F.; Jakobsen, A. L., Eds. *The Routledge Handbook of Translation and Cognition*; Routledge, 2020.
Croucher, S. M.; Cronn-Mills, D. *Understanding Communication Research Methods: A Theoretical and Practical Approach*, 1st ed.; Routledge, 2014.
Mellinger, C.; Hanson, T. *Quantitative Research Methods in Translation and Interpreting Studies*; Routledge, 2016.
Montalt, V.; González-Davies, M. *Medical Translation Step by Step: Learning by Drafting*; Routledge, 2014.
Muñoz-Miquel, A. *La traducción médico-sanitaria: profesión y formación*; Granada: Comares, 2023.
O'Hagan, M., Ed. *The Routledge Handbook of Translation and Technology*; Routledge, 2019.
Pillière, L.; Albachten, Ö. B., Eds. *The Routledge Handbook of Intralingual Translation*; Taylor & Francis, 2024.
Saldanha, G.; O'Brien, S. *Research Methodologies in Translation Studies*; Routledge, 2014.
Susam-Saraeva, Ş.; Spišiaková, E., Eds. *The Routledge Handbook of Translation and Health*; Routledge, 2021.

Thompson, T. L.; Parrott, R.; Nussbaum, J. F., Eds. *The Routledge Handbook of Health Communication*; Routledge, 2011.
Whaley, B. B., Ed. *Research Methods in Health Communication: Principles and Application*; Routledge, 2014.
Williams, J.; Chesterman, A. *The Map: A Beginner's Guide to Doing Research in Translation Studies*; Routledge, 2014.
Wittenberg, E., et al. *Textbook of Palliative Care Communication*, Online ed., Oxford Academic: Oxford; New York, 2015 (accessed Jan 23, 2024).
Zanettin, F.; Rundle, C., Eds. *The Routledge Handbook of Translation and Methodology*; Routledge, 2022.

7.3.2 Research journals

Research journals play a crucial role in advancing the field of patient-centred communication. They serve as platforms for researchers to share their findings and contribute to the existing body of knowledge. Updated research published in journals becomes the foundational reference for future studies as well as a basis for the literature review in any piece of new academic research. Here are some examples that can serve as a starting point:

- *European Journal of Health Communication* (https://ejhc.org/)
- *Communication and Medicine* (https://journal.equinoxpub.com/CAM/about)
- *Health Communication* (www.tandfonline.com/journals/hhth20)
- *International Journal of Person-Centered Medicine* (www.ijpcm.org/index.php/ijpcm)
- *Journal of Communication in Healthcare* (www.tandfonline.com/journals/ycih20)
- *Journal of Health Communication* (www.tandfonline.com/journals/uhcm20)
- *Medical Humanities* (*https://mh.bmj.com/*)
- *Patient Education and Counseling* (www.sciencedirect.com/journal/patient-education-and-counseling)
- *The Journal of Participatory Medicine* (https://jopm.jmir.org/)
- Panace@ (www.tremedica.org/revista-panacea/indice/)
- FITISPos (https://fitisposij.web.uah.es/OJS/index.php/fitispos)
- *Qualitative Health Communication* (https://tidsskrift.dk/qhc)
- *Revista Española de Comunicación en Salud* (https://e-revistas.uc3m.es/index.php/RECS/index)

7.3.3 Databases and social networks

There are several databases that researchers in the field of patient-centred care can use to conduct their literature searches. These databases provide access to a wide range of literature on patient-centred care, including research studies, review articles and other types of publications. It is important for researchers to use a variety of databases to ensure that they are capturing all the relevant literature on their topic of interest. Here are some of the main ones, starting with the more general and moving towards the more specialised:

- Web of Science: Web of Science is another interdisciplinary database that covers a wide range of subject areas, including health sciences. https://access.clarivate.com
- Scopus: Scopus is a large, interdisciplinary database that covers a wide range of subject areas, including health sciences. www.scopus.com/home.uri
- Google scholar http://scholar.google.com
- PubMed www.bing.com/ck/
- CINAHL: The Cumulative Index to Nursing and Allied Health Literature is a database focused on nursing and allied health topics, and it includes articles, books, dissertations and conference proceedings. www.ebsco.com/products/research-databases/cinahl-database
- Cochrane Library: The Cochrane Library is a collection of databases containing high-quality, independent evidence to inform health care decision-making. It includes systematic reviews, clinical trials, and other types of evidence. www.cochranelibrary.com/
- PsycINFO: This database is focused on psychology and related fields and includes articles, books, and dissertations. www.ebsco.com/
- Health and Psychosocial Instruments (HaPI). Produced by Behavioral Measurement Database Services, this bibliographic database is abstracted from hundreds of leading journals in the health and social sciences. HaPI provides comprehensive information about behavioural measurement tools, including those related to medicine and nursing, as well as clinical, personality, social, and developmental psychology. www.ebsco.com/products/research-databases/health-and-psychosocial-instruments-hapi

Last but not least, social networks can be useful for finding researchers and their research in the field of patient-centred communication. Of particular interest are ResearchGate (www.researchgate.net/) and Academia (www.academia.edu/).

GLOSSARY

Accessibility Accessibility refers to the practice of designing products, services, environments and information in a way that is usable by everyone including people with physical, sensory, cognitive and intellectual disabilities.

Ableism and ableist language Ableism is the discrimination against and the systemic exclusion of people with disability. It is often expressed and reinforced through language that is offensive, derogatory, abusive or negative about disability.

Affective communication Affective communication refers to the expression and understanding of emotions in communication. It goes beyond the literal meaning of words and focuses on the emotional undertones. This type of communication plays a crucial role in building relationships, fostering trust and creating a positive environment.

Anamnesis Anamnesis is the process of obtaining information from a patient about the reason for the consultation: the patient's personal and family history, potentially harmful habits and general lifestyle. This information is used to help the doctor diagnose the patient's condition and develop a treatment plan.

Audiodescription A tool for making visual media accessible to blind and partially sighted people. It involves orally narrating key visual elements alongside the existing dialogue and sound effects, creating a richer and more inclusive experience.

Ayurvedic medicine Ayurvedic medicine is one of the world's oldest medical systems and remains one of India's traditional health care systems. It's a holistic approach that emphasizes the balance between mind, body and spirit. Ayurvedic treatment combines products (mainly derived from plants but can include animal, metal and mineral), diet, exercise and lifestyle.

Coherence The quality of a text or discourse being logically interconnected so that it forms a meaningful whole. Transitions, cause-and-effect relationships and overall structure all contribute to coherence. Coherence relies on both the writer/speaker's and the audience's shared knowledge and assumptions about the world. This allows them to make inferences and fill in any gaps left unsaid.

Cohesion The use of grammatical and lexical devices (e.g. pronouns, ellipsis, synonyms, conjunctions) to connect and bind the elements of a text together, creating a meaningful and unified whole; the glue that holds sentences and paragraphs together, ensuring smooth flow, clarity and coherence for the reader.

Collocation The tendency of certain words to co-occur more often than chance alone. These combinations create natural-sounding and idiomatic expressions (e.g. *bitter cold, once in a blue moon*), conveying specific meanings beyond the sum of their individual parts. Understanding and using collocations effectively is crucial for speaking and writing fluently and naturally.

Cluster In corpus linguistics, a cluster refers to a group or set of words, phrases or linguistic items that frequently co-occur within a specific context or pattern across a corpus.

Concordance In corpus linguistics, a concordance is a specialised index that provides a detailed listing of all occurrences of a particular word, phrase or sequence within a corpus.

Cultural competence The ability to interact and communicate effectively with people from diverse cultural backgrounds. It involves understanding, respecting and valuing the beliefs, languages, traditions and norms of different cultural groups. Culturally competent individuals and organisations are able to navigate and bridge cultural differences to promote understanding, inclusivity and equity. They can also improve health outcomes and quality of care and contribute to eliminating racial and ethnic health disparities.

Deixis The phenomenon in language where certain words or phrases depend on contextual information for their interpretation. Thus, a deictic expression or deixis is a word or phrase (such as *this, that, these, those, now, then, here*) that refers to the time, place or situation in which a speaker is speaking or a writer is writing.

Determinologisation De-terminologisation encompasses two interconnected processes. First, it is the practice of replacing technical terminology with accessible language, such as popular synonyms, definitions, analogies or examples, to ensure clarity and comprehension when addressing lay audiences (e.g. *myocardial infarction* replaced by *heart attack*). Secondly, it describes the phenomenon whereby specialised terminology gains wider popularity and moves beyond its original expert contexts, becoming integrated into general public discourse (e.g. *herd immunity, viral variants*).

Discourse community A discourse community is a group of individuals who share a common interest, purpose or goal and who communicate and interact with each other using their own language, terminology and conventions. Examples of discourse communities include academic disciplines (e.g. cardiology, neurology), professional fields (e.g. biomedical research, health care) or social groups (e.g. patient associations).

Ellipsis The omission of one or more words from a sentence or clause that can be understood from contextual clues; ellipsis occurs when a speaker or writer omits certain words that are redundant or predictable, relying on the listener or reader to infer the missing elements.

Ethical competence The ability to understand, recognise and deal effectively and responsibly with ethical dilemmas or challenges. Ethical competence involves having the knowledge, skills and awareness necessary to evaluate ethical issues, make informed decisions and act ethically in professional, personal and social contexts. It can help health care professionals find the best possible solution for patients and is thereby an essential component of high-quality care.

Euphemism A linguistic device used to replace harsh, rude or uncomfortable language with milder or more socially acceptable expressions. It is used to soften the impact of potentially offensive or taboo subjects (such as disability, sex, excretion, or death), maintain social harmony and avoid offence. In addition to these uses, in health care, euphemisms are also used to convey sensitive information such as when breaking bad news, reducing stigma and anxiety or maintaining hope and encouragement in critical situations.

Functionalism An approach in linguistics that focuses on the practical function of language in communication and cognition, as well as its role in shaping social and cultural contexts. It focuses on how language is used in real-life situations, emphasising its communicative and cognitive functions rather than just its formal structure. Functionalists argue that linguistic structures are motivated by their usefulness in facilitating communication and expressing meaning. Overall, functionalism sees language as a dynamic and adaptive system that serves the needs of its users in specific contexts.

Genre (or text genre) Categories of texts that share similar purposes, structures and conventions. These categories help to classify and analyse texts based on their function, content and form. Each genre has its own linguistic features that are used to achieve specific communicative goals within social and cultural contexts. The study of genre involves analysing how language is used to create meaning and achieve purposes in different types of texts and how genres vary across cultures and communities.

Genre competence A communicator's ability to understand and produce texts or utterances in different genres effectively. It involves not only recognising the conventions, structures and purposes of different genres but also knowing how to adapt language use to meet the demands of different communicative contexts. Genre competence encompasses skills such as genre recognition, genre production and genre management that enable speakers to navigate different communicative situations with ease and effectiveness.

Genre shift Also known as *heterofunctional* or *transgeneric* translation; the transformation of a text from one genre to another within the same language or between different languages. This process involves adapting the content, style and linguistic features of the original text to the conventions and expectations of the target genre, for example, transforming an original article into a summary for patients.

Graphic medicine Combines comics or graphic novels with the field of medicine, using visual storytelling to convey medical information, personal experiences of illness, and broader social and ethical issues related to health. It serves purposes such as educating patients, training health care providers, raising awareness of health issues and providing insights into the human experience of illness and healing.

Health literacy The ability of individuals to understand, evaluate and use health information to make informed decisions about their health. It encompasses a range of skills such as reading, listening and critical thinking about health. Improved health literacy enables individuals to navigate health systems effectively, understand medical instructions and adopt healthy behaviours.

Homeopathy A system of alternative medicine developed in the late 18th century by Samuel Hahnemann, a German physician. It is based on the principle that 'like cures like', using highly diluted substances to stimulate the body's natural healing processes. It remains a choice for people seeking alternative or complementary treatments for various health conditions.

Ideology A system of beliefs that offers an interpretation of how the world works and prescribes how it should function, influencing both individual and collective behaviour and identity. It acts as a perceptual lens through which individuals perceive and interact with society, shaping their understanding of and engagement with social structures and norms. Ideological beliefs are deeply embedded in the cultural fabric of a society, and language acts as the primary medium through which these beliefs are articulated, transmitted and perpetuated across generations. Thus, language serves as both a reflection and a vehicle of ideology, shaping the collective consciousness and worldview of a community.

Idiolect A term used in sociolinguistics to refer to the unique linguistic repertoire or speech patterns associated with an individual person. It encompasses the distinctive ways in which an individual uses language, including vocabulary choices, grammatical structures, pronunciation and communication style. Idiolects are shaped by a variety of factors such as upbringing, education, social environment, personal experiences and linguistic influences from peers and the media.

Inclusivity The practice of ensuring that all individuals feel valued, respected and included regardless of their differences or backgrounds. In patient-centred translation and communication, inclusivity ensures that all patients have equal access to health information and services. This includes translating materials into languages that patients understand, providing culturally appropriate resources and involving patients in decision-making. The goal is to create a health care environment where all patients feel valued, respected and empowered to participate in their care.

Inclusive communication Designing messages and interactions that embrace diversity and promote equity, ensuring that everyone, regardless of background or identity, feels respected, valued and included; using language and imagery that is accessible and respectful to all, taking into account different perspectives, cultural sensitivities and cultural differences.

Interactiveness The degree of engagement and responsiveness within a communication process or system. In patient-centred translation and communication, interactiveness refers to the degree to which patients are actively engaged in the communication process. It involves promoting a dynamic exchange of information, feedback and questions between health care providers and patients, as well as among patients themselves. Interactive communication allows patients to express their concerns, preferences and needs while enabling health care providers to respond in a personalised and empathic way.

Intertextuality (referential and functional) In health discourse, the ways in which health and medical texts refer to, borrow from or are influenced by other texts. This can include academic literature citing previous research, health professionals referring to clinical guidelines or case studies, or popular media discussing health-related issues. Intertextuality enables the exchange of knowledge, ideas and practices within the field, enriching understanding and facilitating collaboration. It also highlights the interconnectedness of health-related texts and their dependence on existing research, theories and cultural narratives. In *referential intertextuality*, one text directly refers to, quotes or cites another text; *functional intertextuality* refers to the ways in which texts within a particular discourse or field serve specific functions or purposes by referencing, adapting or responding to other texts.

Intralingual translation Also known as rewriting or paraphrasing, the process of translating text from one language into the same language while retaining the original meaning. It is used to clarify, simplify or adapt content for different audiences within the same linguistic context. It plays a crucial role in improving comprehension, accessibility and effective communication in a variety of fields and contexts, including health care.

Jargon Language used by members of the same profession, social group or academic discipline that is incomprehensible and meaningless to outsiders. A distinction must be made between jargon and technical terminology: unlike technical terminology, which is generally accepted and standardised within a field, jargon may include informal, slang or colloquial expressions that are unique to a particular group or context.

Literacy Includes both basic and functional literacy, which extends reading skills to practical contexts. Critical literacy promotes the ability to analyse and evaluate texts critically, while digital literacy enables individuals to navigate and engage effectively with digital technologies. Information literacy enables the identification, evaluation and responsible use of information from a variety of sources, while media literacy enables individuals to critically analyse and engage with media messages. Finally, cultural literacy is the understanding of shared cultural symbols and traditions.

Together, these dimensions of literacy are essential for individuals to participate fully in society, shaping their ability to make informed decisions, think critically and communicate effectively in an increasingly complex and interconnected world.

Metonymy A linguistic concept whereby an expression symbolises something closely related to its intended meaning. For example, saying "counting heads" instead of people. Although metonyms may seem illogical if taken literally, they're common and follow patterns such as using a place for an event or a part for a whole. Although they may violate semantic constraints, they effectively convey meaning through association and context.

Move (or rhetorical move) A distinct unit or section within a text – a building block of a certain type of writing – that serves a specific communicative function and contributes to the overall coherence of the genre, like research articles or news reports. Each move fulfils a specific function within the genre, such as introducing the topic, establishing the objective, presenting research findings or concluding an argument.

Multimodality The use of multiple modes or forms of communication in a single context or message. Rather than relying solely on written or spoken words, multimodal communication incorporates elements such as images or sounds to convey meaning and provide a richer and more nuanced experience. It's not just about what you say but also how you present it across various sensory channels. For example, some mental health awareness initiatives provide podcasts, video testimonials and online support groups in addition to written information to create a safe space for discussion and resource sharing.

Multiculturalism The presence and interaction of diverse cultures within a society, emphasizing respect, understanding and equal treatment for all groups; goes beyond just acknowledging differences to involve actively embracing and appreciating them.

N-gram In corpus linguistics, an n-gram refers to a contiguous sequence of n items (or words) within a given text or corpus of texts; can be words, letters or other linguistic units, depending on the context and the aims of the analysis.

Neural mirror system A group of specialised neurons that 'mirror' the actions and behaviour of others. The involvement of the mirror neuron system has been implicated in neurocognitive functions (social cognition, language and empathy) and neuropsychiatric disorders.

Paralinguistic aspects The non-verbal elements of communication that accompany spoken language, including tone, pitch, volume, intonation, rhythm and body language. These cues complement verbal communication by conveying emotions, attitudes, emphasis and intentions and are crucial to understanding the full context of a message.

Pluralism Medical pluralism refers to the coexistence and concurrent use of multiple medical systems, practices, or approaches within a society or community. It acknowledges that different cultures and individuals may have diverse beliefs, values, and preferences regarding health and healing, leading them to seek and utilize a variety of medical traditions and therapies. Medical pluralism is a crucial concept in multicultural societies.

Patronising language Speech or writing that conveys an attitude of superiority, condescension or belittlement towards the listener or reader. It typically involves speaking down to someone, assuming that they are less knowledgeable or capable, and may involve using overly simplistic language or tone. Patronising language can reflect paternalistic attitudes and values against patient autonomy. Some phrases or expressions – such as "what we call", "we doctors" – that identify the patient as an outsider who will not understand the information in the text can be particularly patronising.

Pragmatic intentionality The deliberate and purposeful nature of human communication, where writers and speakers use language strategically to convey meaning and achieve desired outcomes in specific social contexts; involves considering the writer's and speaker's intentions, the audience's expectations and the situational context in order to communicate effectively and achieve social goals.

Register Specific linguistic features such as vocabulary, tone and style that are appropriate for a particular communicative setting (social situation, context, purpose, etc.). Registers can vary based on factors like formality, familiarity of participants and subject matter.

***Skopos* theory** A prominent functionalist approach in translation studies that emphasizes the purpose of a translation as the key determinant of its strategies and decisions. The primary consideration is not faithfulness to the source text but achieving the desired *skopos*, which is the aim or function of the translated text in the target culture.

Synonymy Using different words or phrases to have similar meanings or express the same or nearly the same idea. While synonyms may seem like straightforward substitutes, understanding their subtleties can be more complex. While many close matches exist, finding words with identical meanings and contexts is a challenge. Choosing synonyms often involves subtle differences in connotation, register, formality or emphasis.

Tenor The relationship between the participants in a communication event and the social setting in which it occurs; involves looking at factors such as the formality of language, politeness and the use of address forms in different social contexts.

Terminological density A measure of how much terminology related to a specific field or subject is present in the language used; usually refers to the concentration or abundance of technical terms in a piece of text or discourse. High terminological density often indicates a more technical or academic nature and may require a certain level of expertise or familiarity with the subject matter to fully understand it. Low terminological density implies more general or accessible language with fewer specialised terms.

BIBLIOGRAPHY

Adami, E. Multimodality. In *The Oxford Handbook of Language and Society*; García, O.; Flores, N.; Spotti, M., Eds.; Oxford University Press: Oxford, 2017; pp. 451–472.

Agency for Healthcare Research and Quality. *Use the Teach-Back Method: Tool #5*; Agency for Healthcare Research and Quality: Rockville; 2020.

Aleixandre Benavent, R.; Albelda Viana, R.; Ferrer Casanova, C.; Carsí Villalba, E.; Pastor Barberá, J. A.; Cervera Moscardó, J. B. Uso y Abuso de Abreviaturas y Siglas Entre Atención Primaria, Especializada y Hospitalaria. *Papeles Médicos*, 2006, *15* (2), 29–37.

Angelelli, C. V. *Medical Interpreting and Cross-Cultural Communication*; Cambridge University Press: Cambridge, 2008.

Angelelli, C. V. *Studies on Translation and Multilingualism: Study on Public Service Translation in Cross-Border Healthcare*; European Comission. Directorate General for Translation. Publications Office, 2015.

Aragonés, M. *Estudio descriptivo multilingüe del resumen de patente: aspectos contextuales y retóricos*, 1st ed.; Pater Lang: Bern, 2009.

Bakhtin, M. M. *Speech Genres and Other Late Essays*; University of Texas Press: Texas, 1986.

Bazerman, C. Speech Acts, Genres, and Activity Systems: How Texts Organize Activity and People. In *What Writing Does and How It Does It*; Routledge: London, 2003; pp. 315–346.

Bazerman, C. Systems of Genres and the Enactment of Social Intentions. *Genre and the New Rhetoric*, 1994, 79101.

Beach, M. C.; Inui, T. Relationship-Centered Care Research Network. Relationship-Centered Care: A Constructive Reframing. *Journal of General Internal Medicine*, 2006, *21*, 3–8.

Bell, A. Language Style as Audience Design. *Language in Society*, 1984, *13* (2), 145–204.

Bellés-Fortuño, B.; García-Izquierdo, I. Empathic Communication in Healthcare. In *A Multicultural Setting. In Multidisciplinary and Multicultural Discourses: Research and Profession*; Bellés-Fortuño, B., Ed.; Vernon Press: Málaga, Forthcoming.

Berkman, N. D.; Davis, T. C.; McCormack, L. Health Literacy: What Is It? *Journal of Health Communication*, 2010, *15* (Sup 2), 9–19.

Bernardo, M. O.; Cecílio-Fernandes, D.; Costa, P.; Quince, T. A.; Costa, M. J.; Carvalho-Filho, M. A. Physicians' Self-Assessed Empathy Levels Do Not Correlate with Patients' Assessments. *PLoS ONE*, 2018, *13* (5), e0198488.

Bhatia, V. K. *Analysing Genre: Language Use in Professional Settings*, 2nd ed.; Routledge: London, 1993, 2014.

Bhatia, V. K. *Worlds of Written Discourse: A Genre-Based View*, 1st ed.; Continuum: London, 2014.

Biber, D. *Dimensions of Register Variation: A Cross-Linguistic Comparison*; Cambridge University Press: Cambridge; New York, 1995.

Biber, D.; Conrad, S. *Register, Genre, and Style*, 2nd ed.; Cambridge Textbooks in Linguistics; Cambridge University Press: Cambridge; New York, 2019.

Booth, W. C.; Colomb, G. G.; Williams, J. M. *The Craft of Research*, 3rd ed.; Chicago Guides to Writing, Editing, and Publishing; University of Chicago Press: Chicago, 2008.

Borja Albi, A.; García-Izquierdo, I.; Montalt, V. Research Methodology in Specialized Genres for Translation Purposes. *The Interpreter and Translator Trainer*, 2009, *3* (1), 57–77.

Braithwaite, J.; Westbrook, M. T.; Mallock, N. A.; Travaglia, J. F.; Iedema, R. A. Experiences of Health Professionals Who Conducted Root Cause Analyses after Undergoing a Safety Improvement Programme. *BMJ Quality & Safety*, 2006, *15* (6), 393–399.

British Medical Association. *Everyday Medical Ethics and Law*, 1st ed.; Wiley: Blackwell, 2013.

Brown, J.; Noble, L. M.; Papageorgiou, A.; Kidd, J., Eds. *Clinical Communication in Medicine*, 1st ed.; Wiley, 2015.

Byrne, J. *Scientific and Technical Translation Explained: A Nuts and Bolts Guide for Beginners*; Routledge: London, 2014.

Campos Andrés, O. Procedimientos de desterminologización: traducción y redacción de guías para pacientes. *Panace@*, 2013, *14* (37), 48–52.

Carr, B. I. *Understanding Liver Cancer A Tale of Two Diseases*, 1st ed.; Springer Healthcare; Springer, 2014.

Cella, D.; Hahn, E. A.; Jensen, S. E.; Butt, Z.; Nowinski, C. J.; Rothrock, N.; Lohr, K. N. Types of Patient-Reported Outcomes. *Research Triangle Park (NC)*; 2015. https://www.ncbi.nlm.nih.gov/books/NBK424379/.

Chalamon, I.; Chouk, I.; Heilbrunn, B. Does the Patient Really Act Like a Supermarket Shopper? Proposal of a Typology of Patients' Expectations Towards the Healthcare System. *International Journal of Healthcare Management*, 2013, *6* (3), 142–151.

Chall, J. *Readability: An Appraisal of Research and Application*, 1st ed.; Educational Research Monograph; Ohio State Universitty: Columbus, 1958.

Charon, R. Narrative Medicine A Model for Empathy, Reflection, Profession, and Trust. *JAMA*, 2001, *286* (15), 1897–1902.

Ciapuscio, G. E. Formulation and Reformulation Procedures in Verbal Interaction Between Experts and (Semi-) Laypersons. *Discourses Studies*, 2003, *5* (2), 207–233.

Cook-Gumperz, J.; Gumperz, J. Context in Children's Talk. In *The Development of Children's Language*; Waterson Snow, N. C., Ed.; John Wiley: London; New York, 1976; pp. 3–25.

Couper-Kuhlen, E. Comparing Language Use in Social Interaction. In *Studies in Comparative Pragmatics*; Lenk, H. E.; Härmä, J.; Sanromán Vilas, B.; Suomela-Härmä, E., Eds.; Cambridge Scholars Publishing, 2019; pp. 3–18.

Couper-Kuhlen, E.; Selting, M. *Interactional Linguistics: Studying Language in Social Interaction*; Cambridge University Press: Cambridge, 2017.

Crezee, I. H. M. *Introduction to Healthcare for Interpreters and Translators*; John Benjamins Publishing Company: Amsterdam; Philadelphia, 2013.

Crezee, I. H. M.; Road, C. E. Bilingual patient navigator or healthcare interpreter: What's the difference and why does it matter? *Cogent Medicine*, 2019, *6* (1), 181087776.

CRIT. *Culturas y atención sanitaria: guía para la comunicación y la mediación intercultural*; Octaedro; Universitat Jaume I: Barcelona; Castelló, 2009.

Crocker, A. F.; Smith, S. N. Person-First Language: Are We Practicing What We Preach? *JMDH*, 2019, *12*, 125–129. https://doi.org/10.2147/JMDH.S140067.

Dale, E; Chall, J. S. The Concept of Readability. *Elementary English*, 1949, *26* (1), 19–26.

De Linde, Z.; Kay, N. Processing Subtitles and Film Images: Hearing vs Deaf Viewers. *The Translator*, 1999, *5* (1).

Dean, M.; Street, R. L. Patient-Centered Communication. In *Textbook of Palliative Care Communication*; Wittenberg, E.; Ferrell, B. R.; Goldsmith, J.; Smith, T.; Glajchen, M.; Handzo, T. R. G. F., Eds.; Oxford University Press, 2015; pp. 238–245.

Delàs, J., Ed. *Quaderns de la Bona Praxi. Informes clínics, eines de comunicació*; Vol. 18; Col·legi Oficial de Metges de Barcelona: Barcelona, 2005.

Derksen, F.; Bensing, J.; Lagro-Janssen, A. Effectiveness of Empathy in General Practice: A Systematic Review. *British Journal of General Practice*, 2013, *63* (606), e76–e84.

Derksen, F. A. W. M.; Olde Hartman, T.; Bensing, J.; Lagro-Janssen, A. Empathy in General Practice – The Gap between Wishes and Reality: Comparing the Views of Patients and Physicians. *Family Practice*, 2018, *35* (2), 203–208.

Dicciomed: Diccionario médico-biológico, histórico y etimológico. https://dicciomed.usal.es/palabra/arabinosa (accessed Mar 19, 2022).

Díez-Domingo, J.; Fons-Martínez, J.; García-Bayarri, J.; Calvo Rigual, F.; Petrova Dobreva, D.; Vázquez-Moreno, M.; Morales Cuenca, V.; Ferrer-Albero, C.; Egea-Ferrer, M.; García Gómez, A., et al. *Guidelines for Tailoring the Informed Consent Process in Clinical Studies*; Zenodo, 2021.

Domènech-Bagaria, O.; Estopà, R.; Vidal-Sabanés, L. La comprensió dels informes mèdics. In *L'informe mèdic: com millorar-ne la redacció per facilitar-ne la comprensió*, Vol. 47; Estopà, R., Ed.; Fundació Dr. Antoni Esteve: Barcelona, 2020; pp. 28–45.

Drewniak, D.; Glässel, A.; Hodel, M.; Biller-Andorno, N. Risks and Benefits of Web-Based Patient Narratives: Systematic Review. *Journal of Medical Internet Research*, 2020, *22* (3), e15772.

Du Pré, A.; Foster, E. Transactional Communication. In *Textbook of Palliative Care Communication*; Wittenberg, E.; Ferrell, B. R.; Goldsmith, J.; Smith, T.; Glajchen, M.; Handzo, T. R. G. F., Eds.; Oxford University Press, 2015; pp. 14–21.

Dubay, W. *The Principles of Readability*, 1st ed.; Impact Information: CA, 2004.

Edlins, M.; Dolamore, S. Ready to Serve the Public? The Role of Empathy in Public Service Education Programs. *Journal of Public Affairs Education*, 2018, *24* (3), 300–320.

Eggins, S. *An Introduction to Systemic Functional Linguistics*, 2nd ed.; Continuum: New York, 2004.

Engel, G. L. The Need for a New Medical Model: A Challenge for Biomedicine. *Science*, 1977, *196* (4286), 129–136. https://doi.org/10.1126/science.847460.

Epstein, R. M.; Franks, P.; Fiscella, K.; Shields, C. G.; Meldrum, S. C.; Kravitz, R. L.; Duberstein, P. R. Measuring Patient-Centered Communication in Patient–Physician Consultations: Theoretical and Practical Issues. *Social Science & Medicine*, 2005, *61* (7), 1516–1528.

Epstein, R. M.; Street, R. L. *Patient-Centered Communication in Cancer Care: Promoting Healing and Reducing Suffering*; National Cancer Institute: Bethesda, 2007.
Estopà, R., Ed. *L'informe mèdic: com millorar-ne la redacció per facilitar-ne la comprensió*, Vol. 47; Fundació Dr. Antoni Esteve: Barcelona, 2020.
Estopà, R.; Domènech-Bagaria, O. Diagnóstico Del Nivel de Comprensión de Informes Médicos Dirigidos a Pacientes y Familias Afectados Por Una Enfermedad Rara. *E-Aesla*, 2019, *5*, 109–118.
Estopà, R.; Montané, M. A. La terminologia en els informes mèdics. In *L'informe mèdic: com millorar-ne la redacció per facilitar-ne la comprensió*, Vol. 47; Estopà, R., Ed.; Fundació Dr. Antoni Esteve: Barcelona, 2020; pp. 46–59.
European Comission. *Communication from the Commission to the European Parliament, the Council, the European Economic and Social Committee and the Committee of the Regions on Enabling the Digital Transformation of Health and Care in the Digital Single Market*; Empowering Citizens and Building a Healthier Society; 2018.
European Comission. *eHealth Action Plan 2012–2020 – Innovative Healthcare for the 21st Century*; European Comission: Brussels, 2012.
European Comission. *Green Paper on Mobile Health ("mHealth")*; European Comission: Brussels, 2014.
European Union. EU Directive 2001/83/EC; 2001.
Ezpeleta, P. An Example of Genre Shift in the Medicinal Product Information Genre System. *Linguistica Antverpiensia*, 2012, *11*, 167–187.
Fage-Butler, A. M.; Jensen, M. N. Patient- and Family-Centered Written Communication in the Palliative Care Setting. In *Textbook of Palliative Care Communication*; Wittenberg, E.; Ferrell, B. R.; Goldsmith, J.; Smith, T.; Glajchen, M.; Handzo, T. R. G. F., Eds.; Oxford University Press, 2015; pp. 102–110.
Fage-Butler, A. Package Leaflets for Medication in the EU: The Possibility of Integrating Patients' Perspectives in a Regulated Genre? *Medical Writing*, 2015, *24* (4), 210–214.
Farr, J. N.; Jenkins, J. J.; Paterson, D. G. Simplification of Flesch Reading Ease Formula. *Journal of Applied Psychology*, 1951, *35* (3), 333.
Firth, J. R. The Use and Distribution of Certain English Sounds. *English Studies*, 1935, *17* (1–6), 8–18.
Fisher, W. R. *Human Communication as Narration: Toward a Philosophy of Reason, Value, and Action*; University of South Carolina Press: Columbia, 1987.
Fisher, W. R. Clarifying the Narrative Paradigm. *Communications Monographs*, 1989, *56* (1), 55–58.
Flesch, R. *The Art of Readable Writing*, 1st ed.; Harper, 1949.
García-Izquierdo, I. *Divulgación médica y traducción. El género Información para pacientes*; Peter Lang: Bern, 2009.
García-Izquierdo, I. El género: Plataforma de confluencia de nociones fundamentales en didáctica de la traducción. *Discursos*, 2002, 2, 49–63.
García-Izquierdo, I. Investigating Professional Languages through Genres. In *Interdisciplinarity and Languages: Current Issues in Research, Teaching and Professional Applications and ICT*; Selected Papers, Contemporary Studies in Descriptive Linguistics; Peter Lang: Bern, 2011; pp. 125–135.
García-Izquierdo, I.; Montalt, V. Equigeneric and Intergeneric Translation in Patient-Centred Care. *Hermes – Journal of Language and Communication in Business*, 2013, *51*, 39–54.
García-Izquierdo, I.; Montalt, V. Understanding and Enhancing Comprehensibility in Text for Patients in an Institutional Health Care Context in Spain. *RESLA: Special Issue: Specialised Translation in Spain. Institutional Dimensions*, 2017, *30* (2), 592–611.

García-Izquierdo, I.; Montalt, V. Cultural Competence and the Role of the Patient's Mother Tongue: An Exploratory Study of Health Professionals' Perceptions. *Societies*, 2022, *12* (2), 53.
García-Izquierdo, I.; Muñoz-Miquel, A. Los Folletos de Información Oncológica En Contextos Hospitalarios: La Perspectiva de Pacientes y Profesionales Sanitarios. *Panace@ Revista de Medicina, Lenguaje y Traducción*, 2015, *16* (42), 225–231.
Goffman, E. *The Presentation of Self in Everyday Life*; Anchor Books, 1959.
Göpferich, S. Comprehensibility Assessment Using the Kalsruhe Comprehensibility Concept. *The Journal of Specialised Translation*, 2009, *11*, 31–53.
Grainger, K.; Mills, S. *Directness and Indirectness Across Cultures*; Palgrave Macmillan: Houndmills; Basingstoke; Hampshire; New York, 2016.
Gumperz, J. J. Contextualization and Understanding. Rethinking Context. *Language as an Interactive Phenomenon*, 1992, *11*, 229–252.
Gumperz, J. J. Language, Communication, and Public Negotiation. In *Anthropology and the Public Interest*; Elsevier, 1976; pp. 273–292.
Gustin, J.; Stowers, K. H.; Von Gunten, C. F. Communication Education for Physicians. In *Textbook of Palliative Care Communication*; Wittenberg, E.; Ferrell, B. R.; Goldsmith, J.; Smith, T.; Glajchen, M.; Handzo, T. R. G. F., Eds.; Oxford University Press, 2015; pp. 355–365.
Gutiérrez, A. M.; Statham, E. E.; Robinson, J. O.; Slashinski, M. J.; Scollon, S.; Bergstrom, K. L.; Street, R. L.; Parsons, D. W.; Plon, S. E.; McGuire, A. L. Agents of Empathy: How Medical Interpreters Bridge Sociocultural Gaps in Genomic Sequencing Disclosures with Spanish-Speaking Families. *Patient Education and Counseling*, 2019, *102* (5), 895–901.
Hafskjold, L.; Sundler, A. J.; Holmström, I. K.; Sundling, V.; van Dulmen, S.; Eide, H. A Cross-Sectional Study on Person-Centred Communication in the Care of Older People: The COMHOME Study Protocol. *BMJ Open*, 2015, *5* (4), e007864. https://doi.org/10.1136/bmjopen-2015-007864.
Hall, E. T. *Beyond Culture*; Anchor Books/Doubleday: New York, 1976.
Hall, E. T. The Power of Hidden Differences. In *Basic Concepts of Intercultural Communication*; Bennett, M. J., Ed.; Intercultural Press Inc.: Maine, 1998; pp. 53–67.
Halliday, M. A. K. Systemic Theory. In *Concise History of the Language Sciences*; Koerner, E. F. K.; Asher, R. E., Eds.; Pergamon, 1995; pp. 272–276.
Halliday, M. A. K.; Hasan, R. *Language, Context, and Text: Aspects of Language in a Social-semiotic Perspective*; Oxford University Press: Oxford, 1985.
Halliday, M. A. K.; Matthiessen, C. M. *Halliday's Introduction to Functional Grammar*; Routledge, 2013.
Halliday, M. A. K.; Webster, J., Eds. *Continuum Companion to Systemic Functional Linguistics*; Continuum: London; New York, 2009.
Hansen, M. M.; Zethsen, K. K. Is Electronic Access to Medical Records an Empowering and Patient-Centered Initiative? – A Qualitative Contextual and Linguistic Analysis of Danish Electronic Records. *HJLCB*, 2018, *58*, 157–173.
Hasan, R. Meaning, Context and Text: Fifty Years After Malinowski. *Systemic Perspectives on Discourse*, 1985, *1*, 16–47.
Hatim, B.; Mason, I. *Discourse and the Translator*; Routledge: London, 1990.
Hatim, B.; Mason, I. *The Translator as Communicator*; Routledge: London, 1997.
Hausberg, M. C.; Hergert, A.; Kröger, C.; Bullinger, M.; Rose, M.; Andreas, S. Enhancing Medical Students' Communication Skills: Development and Evaluation of an Undergraduate Training Program. *BMC Medical Education*, 2012, *12* (1), 16.
Heinemann, L.; Drossel, D.; Freckmann, G.; Kulzer, B. Usability of Medical Devices for Patients With Diabetes Who Are Visually Impaired or Blind. *Journal of Diabetes Science and Technology*, 2016, *10* (6), 1382–1387. https://doi.org/10.1177/1932296816666536.

Hemberg, J.; Sved, E. The Significance of Communication and Care in One's Mother Tongue: Patients' Views. *Nordic Journal of Nursing Research*, 2021, *41* (1), 42–53.

Herber, O. R.; Gies, V.; Schwappach, D.; Thürmann, P.; Wilm, S. Patient Information Leaflets: Informing or Frightening? A Focus Group Study Exploring Patients' Emotional Reactions and Subsequent Behavior towards Package Leaflets of Commonly Prescribed Medications in Family Practices. *BMC Family Practice*, 2014, *15* (1), 163.

Hirsh, D.; Clerehan, R.; Staples, M.; Osborne, R. H.; Buchbinder, R. Patient Assessment of Medication Information Leaflets and Validation of the Evaluative Linguistic Framework (ELF). *Patient Education and Counseling*, 2009, *77* (2), 248–254.

Hua, Z. *Exploring Intercultural Communication: Language in Action*; Routledge Introduction to Applied Linguistics; Routledge: Milton Park; Abingdon; Oxon; New York, 2014.

Iedema, R.; Carroll, K.; Collier, A.; Hor, S. Y.; Mesman, J.; Wyer, M. *Video-Reflexive Ethnography in Health Research and Healthcare Improvement: Theory and Application*; CRC Press, 2019.

Jakobson, R. On Linguistic Aspects of Translation. In *On Translation*; Brower, R. A., Ed.; Harvard University Press, 1959; pp. 232–239.

James, L. C.; Bharadia, T. Lay Summaries and Writing for Patients: Where are We Now and Where Are We Going? *Medical Writing*, 2019, *28* (3), 6.

Jarret C.; Gaffney G. *Forms that Work: Designing Web Forms for Usability*; M K Elsevier: Barlington, 2009.

Jarret, C.; Redish, J. *Readability Formulas: 7 Reasons to Avoid Them and What to Do Instead*; 2019. www.uxmatters.com/mt/archives/2019 (accessed Sep 10, 2021).

Jensen, M. N. Optimising Comprehensibility in Interlingual Translation: The Need for Intralingual Translation. In *Translation and Comprehensibility*; Maksymski, K.; Gutermuth, S.; Hansen-Schirra, S., Eds.; Frank und Timme: Berlin, 2015; pp. 163–194.

Jensen, M. N.; Zethsen, K. K. Lay-Friendliness in Translated Patient Information Leaflets. *International Conference on Communication in Healthcare*; 2011. https://pure.au.dk/ws/files/41561340/Final_poster.pdf.

Jensen, M. N.; Zethsen, K. K. Translation of Patient Information Leaflets: Trained Translators and Pharmacists-Cum-Translators–a Comparison. *Linguistica Antverpiensia, New Series–Themes in Translation Studies*, 2012, *11*, 31–49.

Ji, M.; Taibi, M.; Crezee, I. H. *Multicultural Health Translation, Interpreting and Communication*; Routledge, 2019 (2nd ed., 2021).

Joffe, S.; Truog, R. D. Consent to Medical Care: The Importance of Fiduciary Context. *The Ethics of Consent: Theory and Practice*, 2010, *43* (7), 347–373.

Kalavana, T. V. Responding to Emotions. In *Clinical Communication in Medicine*; Brown, J.; Noble, L. M.; Papageorgiou, A.; Kidd, J., Eds.; Wiley, 2015; pp. 91–97.

Katan, D. Defining Culture, Defining Translation. In *The Routledge Handbook of Translation and Culture*; Harding, S. A.; Cortés, O. C., Eds.; Routledge, 2018; pp. 17–47.

Katan, D.; Taibi, M. *Translating Cultures: An Introduction for Translators, Interpreters and Mediators*; Routledge, 2021.

Khalikova, V. Doctors of Plural Medicine, Knowledge Transmission, and Family Space in India. *Medical Anthropology*, 2020, *39* (3), 282–296.

Khalikova, V. Medical Pluralism. In *The Open Encyclopedia of Anthropology*; Stein, F., Ed.; *Facsimile of the First Edition in The Cambridge Encyclopedia of Anthropology*, 2023. http://doi.org/10.29164/21medplural.

Klare, G. R.; The *Measurement of Readability*; The Iowa State University Press: Ames, Iowa 1963.

Kleinig, J. The Nature of Consent. *The Ethics of Consent: Theory and Practice*, 2010, *3*, 3–24.

Kleinman, A.; Eisenberg, L.; Good, B. Culture, Illness, and Care: Clinical Lessons from Anthropologic and Cross-Cultural Research. *Annals of Internal Medicine*, 1978, *88* (2), 251.

Lang, S.; Esser, M. Improving Patient Communication by Writing with Empathy. *Medical Writing*, 2012, *21* (4), 305–307. https://doi.org/10.1179/2047480612Z.00000000048.

Little, P. Preferences of Patients for Patient Centred Approach to Consultation in Primary Care: Observational Study. *BMJ*, 2001, *322* (7284), 468–468.

Llopart-Saumel, E.; Da Cunha, I. L'Informe mèdic com a gènere textual. In *L'informe mèdic: com millorar-ne la redacció per facilitar-ne la comprensió*, Vol. 47; Estopà, R., Ed.; Fundació Dr. Antoni Esteve: Barcelona, 2020; pp. 32–45.

Maat, H. P.; Lentz, L. Improving the Usability of Patient Information Leaflets. *Patient Education and Counseling*, 2010, *80* (1), 113–119.

Malinowski, B. Psycho-Analysis and Anthropology. *Nature*, 1923, *112* (2818), 650–651.

Marsden, A. J. *Empathetic Consultation Skills in Undergraduate Medical Education: A Qualitative Approach*; University of East Anglia, 2014.

Martin, J. R. *English Text: System and Structure*; Benjamins: Philadelphia, 1992.

Mason, I. Audience Design in Translating. *The Translator*, 2000, *6* (1), 1–22.

Medicines and Healthcare Products Regulatory Agency. *Best Practice Guidance on Patient Information Leaflets*; 2012. https://assets.publishing.service.gov.uk/media/5fe086c18fa8f5149718d66a/Best_practice_guidance_on_patient_information_leaflets.pdf.

Mehlman, M. J. Why Physicians Are Fiduciaries for Their Patients. *Indian. Health Law Review*, 2015, *12* (1), 1–65.

Mogami, S.; Noyes, M.; Morita, R.; Shiotsuki, A.; Hagi, T.; Hasegawa, H.; Kikuchi, C. Creation of a Patient-Centric Patient Lay Summary in the Local Language. *Medical Writing*, 2017, *26*, 42–45.

Montalt, V. Ethical Considerations in the Translation of Health Genres in Crisis Communication. 17. In *Translating Crises*; O'Brien, S.; Federici, F. M., Ed.; Bloomsbury Publishing, 2022; p. 17.

Montalt, V.; Shuttleworth, M. Research in Translation and Knowledge Mediation in Medical and Healthcare Settings. *Linguistica Antverpiensia*, 2012, *11*, 9–30.

Montalt, V. Medical Humanities and Translation. In *The Routledge Handbook of Translation and Health*; Routledge, 2021.

Montalt, V. Patient-Centred Translation and Emerging Trends in Medicine and Health Care. *European Society for Translation Studies (EST) Newsletter*, 2017, *51*, 10–11.

Montalt, V. Researching Informed Consent (IC) – A Translational Perspective. *UCL Research Seminar*. www.ucl.ac.uk/european-languages-culture/events/2022/jan/researching-informed-consent-ic-translational-perspective (accessed Mar 19, 2022).

Montalt, V.; García-Izquierdo, I. Emerging Conceptualizations of Mediation in Medical and Healthcare Settings. *Translation & Interpreting Studies*, 2024, *18* (2).

Montalt, V.; García-Izquierdo, I. Exploring the Links Between the Oral and the Written in Patient–Doctor Communication. In *Medical Discourse in Professional, Academic and Popular Settings*; Ordóñez-López, P.; Edo-Marzá, N., Eds.; Multilingual Matters, 2016b; pp. 103–124.

Montalt, V.; García-Izquierdo, I. ¿Informar o Comunicar? Algunos Temas Emergentes En Comunicación Para Pacientes. *Panace@*, 2016a, *17* (44), 81–84.

Montalt, V.; García-Izquierdo, I. Translating Into Textual Genres. *Linguistica Antverpiensia*, 2002, *1*, 135–145.

Montalt, V.; González Davies, M. *Medical Translation Step by Step: Learning by Drafting*; Translation Practices Explained; Saint Jerome Publishing: Manchester, 2007.

Muñoz-Miquel, A. Bridging the Gap between Professional Practice and University Training through Socio-Professional Research: The Case of Medical Translation. In *From the Lab to the Classroom and Back Again: Perspectives on Translation and Interpreting Training*, Vol. 19; Martín de León, C.; González-Ruiz, V., Eds.; New Trends in Translation Studies; Peter Lang: Oxford, 2016; pp. 257–294.

Muñoz-Miquel, A. *El perfil del traductor médico: análisis y descripción de competencias específicas para su formación.* Tesis doctoral; Universitat Jaume I, 2014.

Muñoz-Miquel, A. Empathy, Emotions and Patient-Centredness: A Case Study on Communication Strategies. *HERMES: Journal of Language and Communication in Business*, 2019, *59* (1), 71–89.

Muñoz-Miquel, A. From the Original Article to the Summary for Patients: Reformulation Procedures in Intralingual Translation. *Linguistica Antverpiensia*, 2012, *11*, 187–206.

Muñoz-Miquel, A.; Ezpeleta-Piorno, P.; Saiz-Hontangas, P. Intralingual Translation in Healthcare Settings: Strategies and Proposals for Medical Translator Training. *MonTI*, 2018, *10*, 177–204.

Munsour, E. E.; Awaisu, A.; Azmi Ahmad Hassali, M.; Darwish, S.; Abdoun, E. Readability and Comprehensibility of Patient Information Leaflets for Antidiabetic Medications. *Journal of Pharmacy Technology*, 2017, *33* (4), 128–136.

Napier, A. D.; Ancarno, C.; Butler, B.; Calabrese, J.; Chater, A.; Chatterjee, H.; Guesnet, F.; Horne, R.; Jacyna, S.; Jadhav, S. Culture and Health. *The Lancet*, 2014, *384* (9954), 1607–1639.

Navarro, F. A. Diccionario de términos médicos de la Real Academia Nacional de Medicina: el sueño de un dermatólogo hecho por fin realidad. *Más Dermatology*, 2012, *17*, 2–4.

Neubauer, K.; Dixon, W.; Corona, R.; Bodurtha, J. Cultural Humility. In *Textbook of Palliative Care Communication*; Wittenberg, E.; Ferrell, B. R.; Goldsmith, J.; Smith, T.; Glajchen, M.; Handzo, T. R. G. F., Eds.; Oxford University Press, 2015; pp. 79–89.

NHS Digital. Professional Record Standards Body; Royal College of Physicians. In *PRSB Standards for the Structure and Content of Health and Care Records*; NHS Digital: London, 2018.

Nord, C. *Translation as a Purposeful Activity, Functionalist Approaches Explained*; St. Jerome Publishing: Manchester, 1997.

O'Brien, S.; Federici, F. M. Crisis Translation: Considering Language Needs in Multilingual Disaster Settings. *Disaster Prevention and Management: An International Journal*, 2019, *29* (2), 129–143.

O'Halloran, K.; Smith, B. A., Eds. *Multimodal Studies: Exploring Issues and Domains*, Vol. 2; Routledge, 2012.

Orlikowski, W. J.; Yates, J. *Genre Repertoire: Norms and Forms for Work and Interaction*; 1994a. www.dspace.mit.edu.

Orlikowski, W. J.; Yates, J. Genre Repertoire: The Structuring of Communicative Practices in Organizations. *Administrative Science Quarterly*, 1994b, *39* (4), 541–574.

Ortí, R.; Sánchez, E.; Sales, D. Interacción Comunicativa En La Atención Sanitaria a Inmigrantes: Diagnóstico de Necesidades (in) Formativas Para La Mediación Intercultural. *Actas del Primer Congreso Nacional de Lingüística Clínica*, 2006, *3*, 114–139.

O'Sullivan, C. Introduction: Multimodality as Challenge and Resource for Translation. *The Journal of Specialised Translation*, 2013, *20*, 2–14.

Parrilla Gómez, L.; Postigo Pinazo, E. Intercultural Communication and Interpreter's Roles: Widening Taxonomies for Effective Interaction within the Healthcare Context. *Current Trends in Translation Teaching and Learning E*, 2018, *5*, 236–314.

Patient-Led Research Collaborative. About the Patient Generated Hypotheses Journal. *Patient-Generated Hypotheses Journal for Long COVID & Associated Conditions*, 2023, *1*, 1–3.

Perdiguero, E. El Fenómeno Del Pluralismo Asistencial: Una Realidad Por Investigar. *Gaceta Sanitaria*, 2004, *18* (supl 1), 140–145.

Pérez Estevan, E. *Interpretación En Final de Vida y Duelo: Un Modelo Psicolingüístico de Análisis Aplicado a Situaciones de Malas Noticias, Últimos Días y Duelo*; Tesis doctoral; Universidad de Alicante; 2022.

Pilegaard, M.; Ravn, H. B. Readability of Patient Information Can Be Improved. *Danish Medical Journal*, 2012, *59* (5), 1–5.

Pons, X. La comunicación entre el profesional de la salud y el paciente: aspectos conceptuales y guías de aplicación. *Enfermería integral*, 2006, *27* (2), 27–34.

Prieto-Velasco, J. A.; Montalt, V. Encouraging Comprehensibility through Multimodal Patient Information Guides. *Linguistica Antverpiensia, New Series – Themes in Translation Studies*, 2018, *17*, 196–214.

Remael, A.; Reviers, N.; Vercauteren, G., Eds. *Pictures Painted in Words ADLAB Audio Description Guidelines*; 2015. www.adlabproject.eu/Docs/adlab%20book/index.html.

Revheim, N.; Corcoran, C. M.; Dias, E; Hellmann, E; Martínez, A; Butler, P.; Lehrfeld, J. M.; DiCostanzo, J; Albert, J; Javitt, D. C. Reading Deficits in Schizophrenia and Individuals at High Clinical Risk: Relationship to Sensory Function, Course of Illness, and Psychosocial Outcome. *American Journal of Psychiatry*, 2014, *171* (9), 949–959.

Ribeiro-Alves, A.; Ferreira Cabrera, A. Estudio de Corpus: Estructura y Legibilidad en el Documento de Consentimiento Informado en el ámbito académico-profesional de las Ciencias Biomédicas. *RLA. Revista de lingüística teórica y aplicada*, 2018, *56* (2), 91–116.

Riessman, C. K. *Narrative Methods for the Human Sciences*; Sage: London, 2008.

Rike, S. M. Bilingual Corporate Websites – from Translation to Transcreation? *Journal of Specialised Translation*, 2013, *20*, 68–85.

Rogers, C. R. *A Way of Being*; Houghton Mifflin Harcourt, 1995.

Romero-Fresco, P. Accessing Communication: The Quality of Live Subtitles in the UK. *Language & Communication*, 2016, *49*, 56–69.

Rønning, S. B.; Bjørkly, S. The Use of Clinical Role-Play and Reflection in Learning Therapeutic Communication Skills in Mental Health Education: An Integrative Review. *Advances in Medical Education and Practice*, 2019, eCollection.

Rosenzweig, M. Q. Breaking Bad News: A Guide for Effective and Empathetic Communication. *The Nurse Practitioner*, 2012, *37* (2), 1–4.

Ruiz Mezcua, A. Interpretación y Formación Para Los Centros Sanitarios Españoles. *Hermēneus. Revista de Traducción e Interpretación*, 2014, *16*, 265–289.

Ruiz-Moral, R.; Pérula De Torres, L.; Monge, D.; García Leonardo, C.; Caballero, F. Teaching Medical Students to Express Empathy by Exploring Patient Emotions and Experiences in Standardized Medical Encounters. *Patient Education and Counseling*, 2017, *100* (9), 1694–1700.

Saiz Hontangas, P.; Ezpeleta-Piorno, P.; Muñoz-Miquel, A. El Uso de Imágenes En Guías Para Pacientes: Una Primera Aproximación Desde La Perspectiva Del Nivel de Activación Del Paciente. *Panace@*, 2016, *44* (17), 99–110.

Semino, E. Metaphor in the Experience of Illness. In *Metaphor in the Experience of Illness*; Universitat Jaume I, 2020.

Semino, E. Not Soldiers but Fire-Fighters – Metaphors and Covid-19. *Health Communication*, 2021, *36* (1), 50–58.

Semino, E.; Demjén, Z., Eds. *The Routledge Handbook of Metaphor and Language*; Routledge Handbooks in Linguistics; Routledge: London; New York, 2017.

Shaw, J. M.; Dunn, S. M.; Heirich, P. Managing the Delivery of Bad New: An In-depth Analysis of Doctors Delivery Style. *Patient Education and Counseling*, 2012, *91*, 243–248.

Shuttleworth, M. *Studying Scientific Metaphor in Translation: An Inquiry into Cross-Lingual Translation Practices*; Routledge Advances in Translation and Interpreting Studies; Routledge; Taylor & Francis Group: New York; London, 2017.

Silverman, J. Relationship Building. In *Clinical Communication in Medicine*; Brown, J.; Noble, L. M.; Papageorgiou, A.; Kidd, J., Eds.; Wiley, 2015; pp. 72–75.

Silverman, J.; Draper, J.; Kurtz, S. M. The Calgary-Cambridge Approach to Communication Skills Teaching 2: The SET-GO Method of Descriptive Feedback. *Education for General Practice*, 1997, *8*, 16–23.

Singh, K.; Landman, A. B. Mobile Health. In *Key Advances in Clinical Informatics*; Elsevier, 2017; pp. 183–196.

Sivanadarajah, N.; El-Daly, I.; Mamarelis, G.; Sohail, M. Z.; Bates, P. Informed Consent and the Readability of the Written Consent Form. *The Annals of The Royal College of Surgeons of England*, 2017, *99* (8), 645–649.

Skelton, J. *Role Play and Clinical Communication: Learning the Game*; Radcliffe Publishing, 2008.

Smith, S. G.; Jackson, S. E.; Kobayashi, L. C.; Steptoe, A. Social Isolation, Health Literacy, and Mortality Risk: Findings from the English Longitudinal Study of Ageing. *Health Psychology*, 2018, *37* (2), 160.

Sontag, S. *La enfermedad y sus metáforas. El sida y sus metáforas*; De Bolsillo: Madrid, 1978.

Sparks, L.; Villagran, M. M.; Parker-Raley, J.; Cunningham, C. B. A Patient-Centered Approach to Breaking Bad News: Communication Guidelines for Health Care Providers. *Journal of Applied Communication Research*, 2007, *35* (2), 177–196.

Spinuzzi, C.; Zachry, M. Genre Ecologies: An Open-System Approach to Understanding and Constructing Documentation. *ACM. Journal of Computer Documentation*, 2000, *24* (3), 169–181.

Suojanen, T.; Koskinen, K.; Tuominen, T. *User-Centered Translation*, First Published; Translation Practices Explained; Routledge: London; New York, 2015.

Swales, J. M. *Genre Analysis: English in Academic and Research Settings*; The Cambridge Applied Linguistics Series; Cambridge University Press: Cambridge; New York, 1990.

Szigriszt Pazos, F. *Readability Predictive Systems of the Written Message: Formula Perspicuity*; Universidad Complutense de Madrid: Madrid, 1993.

Tate, P.; Frame, F. *The Doctor's Communication Handbook*, 8th ed.; Radcliffe Publishing Ltd; CRC Press: London; New York, 2019.

Thompson, T. L.; Harrington, N. G., Eds. *The Routledge Handbook of Health Communication*; Routledge Communication Series, 3rd ed.; Routledge: New York; London, 2022.

Thompson, T. L.; Parrott, R.; Nussbaum, J. F., Eds. *The Routledge Handbook of Health Communication*. Routledge: New York; London, 2011.

Valero Garcés, C.; Alcalde Peñalver, E. Empathy in PSI: Where We Stand and Where to Go from Here. *FITISPos-IJ*, 2021, *8* (1), 17–27.

Vandaele, S. Conceptualisation Indices in Health and Life Sciences Translation: An Experientialist Approach. *MonTI. Monografías De Traducción E Interpretación*, 2018, *10*, 225–256. https://doi.org/10.6035/MonTI.2018.10.9

Vandekieft, G. K. Breaking Bad News. *American Family Physician*, 2001, *64* (12), 1975–1979.

Vedsted, P.; Heje, H. N. Association between Patients' Recommendation of Their GP and Their Evaluation of the GP. *Scandinavian Journal of Primary Health Care*, 2008, *26* (4), 228–234.

Wilkinson, H.; Whittington, R.; Perry, L.; Eames, C. Examining the Relationship between Burnout and Empathy in Healthcare Professionals: A Systematic Review. *Burnout Research*, 2017, *6*, 18–29.

Wolfer, S. Comprehension and Comprehensibility. In *Translation and Comprehensibility*; Frank und Timme: Berlin, 2015; p. 34.

World Health Organization. *Digital Health*. www.who.int/health-topics/digital-health#tab=tab_1 (accessed June 9, 2022).

World Health Organization. *Global Observatory for eHealth*. www.who.int/observatories/global-observatory-for-ehealth.

World Health Organization. *Monitoring Health for the SDGS (Sustainable Development Goals)*; 2016. https://www.who.int/publications/i/item/9789241565264.

Wright, P. Writing and Information Design of Healthcare Materials. In *Writing Texts, Processes and Practices*; Candlin, C.; Hyland, K., Eds.; Routledge, 1999; pp. 85–98.

Yamasaki, J.; Sharf, B. F.; Harter, L. M. Narrative Inquiry. Attitude, Acts, Artifacts, and Analysis. In *Research Methods in Health Communication*; Whaley, B. B., Ed.; Routledge: New York; London, 2014; pp. 99–118.

Yates, J.; Orlikowski, W. Genre Systems: Structuring Interaction through Communicative Norms. *The Journal of Business Communication*, 2002, *39* (1), 13–35.

Young, A.; Tordoff, J.; Smith, A. 'What Do Patients Want?' Tailoring Medicines Information to Meet Patients' Needs. *Research in Social and Administrative Pharmacy*, 2017, *13* (6), 1186–1190.

Zenasni, F.; Boujut, E.; Woerner, A.; Sultan, S. Burnout and Empathy in Primary Care: Three Hypotheses. *British Journal of General Practice*, 2012, *62* (600), 346–347. https://doi.org/10.3399/bjgp12X652193.

Zethsen, K. K. Access Is Not the Same as Understanding. Why Intralingual Translation Is Crucial in a World of Information Overload. *Across Languages and Cultures*, 2018, *19* (1), 79–98.

Zethsen, K. K. Beyond Translation Proper – Extending the Field of Translation Studies. *TTR*, 2007, *20* (1), 281–308.

Zethsen, K. K. Intralingual Translation: An Attempt at Description. *Meta*, 2009, *54* (4), 795–812.

Zethsen, K. K.; Montalt, V. Translating Medical Texts. In *The Cambridge Handbook of Translation*; Malmkjær, K., Ed.; Cambridge University Press: Cambridge, 2022; pp. 363–378.

Zhao, J.; Abrahamson, K.; Anderson, J. G.; Ha, S.; Widdows, R. Trust, Empathy, Social Identity, and Contribution of Knowledge within Patient Online Communities. *Behaviour & Information Technology*, 2013, *32* (10), 1041–1048.

INDEX

Note: Page numbers in *italics* indicate a figure and page numbers in **bold** indicate a table on the corresponding page.

ableism 131; intentional/unintentional 132
ableist language 131–132
accessibility 61, 69, 77, 160; blind and partially sighted patients 69–71; deaf and hard of hearing patients 71–72; and multimodality 158–159; patients with learning difficulties 72–73; research process 158–159
ADLAB/ADLAB PRO projects 70
affective communication 8
Aleixandre Benavent, R. 49
Amazon Alexa 73
anamnesis 53
Annals of Internal Medicine *40*, *41*
anthropology 15, 117
applied linguistics 102, 104, 117
artificial intelligence (AI) 160; medical devices 74
audiences 79–80; active role of 80–81; analysing 92–93; continuum of *91*, *93*; expectations 90; and genres 82–83; lay friendly 91, *92*; and levels of reception 87–90; motivation 90–91; in patient-centred way 98–99; reading process 89; research process 156–157; situation 83–87
audio description (AD) 61, 69, 70
augmented speech 158
ayurvedic medicine 25

Bakhtin, M. M. 81
behaviour change techniques (BCTs) 76
Bell, A. 84
blind and partially sighted patients 69–71
Booth, W. C. 161
Braille 69, 70

Calgary–Cambridge Guide (CCG) 66, 67, 82
Chall, J. S. 101
Chinese medicine 25
clusters 29, 139
Cochrane Library 163
coherence 65, 108, 142
cohesion 16
collocations 37
Colomb, G. G. 161
comic strips 57–59
communication 6, 54; conversation analysis 145; culture, influence of 21; degree of directness 22; degree of explicitness 21–22; fostering skills 67–68; in health care settings 27; high- *vs.* low-context cultures 21–22; inter- and intralingual 159;

medical reports 48; multilingual and multicultural 94; multimodality 158; non-verbal 23, 68, 123; oral 115, 123; paralinguistic aspects 23–24; patient-centredness 8; patients with learning difficulties 72; person-centred approach 7; power distance 22; taboo topics 22–23; technologies 56; of text-mediated 90; verbal 68; written 126–127
communicative exchange 18–19
communicative situation 83; channels 86; communicative purposes 87; participants 83–85; patient-doctor relationship 85; processing circumstances 86; setting 86–87
comparable corpora 139, 154
compassion 116–117; fatigue 119
comprehensibility 88, 100–101; characteristics 101–103; definition 101–103; factors 103–104; Flesch's reading ease scores **107**; improvement 109–114, **111**; lack of 104–106; quantitative measurements 108; readability formulas 106–109; research process 155–156; texts addressed to patients 110–112
concordance 10, 13, 151, 152
context 15–18, 159; AD 70; clinical research 51; clinical trials 53, 82; Covid-19 pandemic 96; of culture 18–19, 83, 142, 150–151; of culture in patient-centred communication 19, 79; educational 146; of genre 28–29; health care 36; health communication 141; health policy 51; high- *vs.* low culture 21–22; IC 43–45; ideological 140; interpreters 124; medical and health care 119; multiculturalism 106; palliative care 147; patient-centred care 102; patient diversity 95; pedagogical 30; PIL 17; pluralism 106; setting 86; of situation 18–19; social 83, 142
contextualisation, concepts of 16, 17
conversation analysis 145, 156
corpus linguistics 139–140
Covid-19 pandemic 30; cultural and ideological attitudes 96; digitalisation 74–76; e-health 61, 74–75; empathy 119; lockdowns 65; Patient-Led Research Collaborative 148
The craft of research (Booth, Colomb and Williams) 161
Crezee, I. 21
critical discourse analysis (CDA) 140–141, 151, 154
cultural diversity 18
culture 6, 7, 10, 123, 155; attitudes 96; communication 20–21; and context 150–151; context of 18–19, 21–22; definition 20–21; degree of directness 22; and degree of explicitness 21–22; in empathy 134; ethnicity/national 156; and health 24–25, 157; health care communication 134; high- *vs.* low-context 21–22; home health care 103; and language 27, 28, 62; literacy level and professional 156; non-verbal communication 23; paralinguistic aspects 23–24; in patient-centred communication 19; power distance 22; research process 150–151; taboo topics 22–23
Cumulative Index to Nursing and Allied Health Literature (CINAHL) 163

Dale, E. 101
deaf and hard of hearing patients 71–72
degree of directness 21, 22
degree of explicitness 21–22
deixis 16
de-terminologisation 16
diabetic ketoacidosis (DKA) 11–12
digitalisation: and e-health 74–75; multimodal genres 75–78
digital patients 74
digital storytelling 54
discourse community 109
disease 32–33, 36; biomedical knowledge of 85; heart 105; Parkinson's 95, 98; physical aspects of 7
doctor-centred approaches 6, 7, 10
dramaturgical analysis 145–146
Dubay, W. H. 101
Du Pré, A. 118

education and training 151–153
e-health 49, 56, 61, 74–75
electronic health records (EHRs) 75–76
ellipsis 31
emotional distress 10, 86, 121–122, 129
emotional intelligence 9
emotional well-being 9, 87
emotions 9, 14, 117; distress 121–122; research process 155–156

empathy 7, 10, 35, 115–116; cultural variation in 134; definition 116–117; in face-to-face interactions 120–125; in fiction 125; lack of 108; in oral communication 119–120; in patient-centred communication 117–119; in written communication 126–134
Engel, G. L. 7
Epocrates® *57*
Esser, M. 127–128
ethical competence 45
euphemism 65, 104, 122, 131
European Commission's report 17
European Union 13, 18, 57
expert-lay translation 109, 126

face-to-face consultations 60, 63, 65, 69; patient-centred care 10; verbal and non-verbal information 62
face-to-face interactions, in empathy 120; eliciting concerns 121–122; emotional distress 121–122; forecasting 122; leaving room for questions 120; listening actively 120; non-verbal communication 123; plural pronouns 121; reasoned explanations 121; self-disclosure to establish trust and rapport 121; simplifying language 122–123; strategies for interpreters 124–125, *123*
fact sheet, patients 27, 32, 33, 52, 109, 129; *vs.* adequacy for patients 38; empathy 134; for patients 36–37; WHO response *37*
Fage-Butler, A. M. 127
false friend 91
Farr, J. N. 107
Firth, J. R. 15–16
Flesch, R. 107; Reading Ease formula 107, 134
focus groups 119, 144, 149, 153, 157
Foster, E. 118
functionalism 102

Garcés, V. 119
genres 16, 19, 20, 27, 60, 153–154; and audiences 82–83; colonies 30; comics 57–59; competence 166; definition 28–29; ecology 30; fact sheet 36–38; GENTT research group *31*, 139; grouping 29–30; health app 56–57; informed consent 43–47; medical report 47–51; patient narratives 53–56; patient-reported outcomes 51–52; patient summaries 39–43; PIL 34–36; repertoires of 29; research process 153–154; shift 109–110, 113–114; systems 29
GENTT research group 46, 120, 123, 127, 129, 140; genre analysis template 30, *31*
Goffman, E. 145
Gómez, P. 123
Google Assistant 73
Google's Bards GPT 160
Google scholar 163
graphic medicine 57, 58
group genres 29–31
Gumperz, J. J. 16
Gutiérrez, A. M. 124

Hall, E. T. 21, 22
Hansen, M. M. 50
Hatim, B. 19
Health and Psychosocial Instruments (HaPI) 163
health app 56–57
health care system 10, 32, 57, 70, 81, 89; beliefs and practices 25; and culture 24–25; effectiveness of 100; machine translation 160; pharmacological treatment 43
health literacy 79, 89, 103, 104
health-related quality of life (HRQoL) 51
Herber, O. R. 126

ideology 19; CDA 140
Iedema, R. 147
illness 6, 10, 14; attitudes 96; chronic 122; focus groups 144; life-threating 22; mental 154; patient's experience of 7, 13, 52, 53–56
inclusive communication 60
inclusivity 61, 69, 158
infertility 24, 118, 121; definition 135
Inflesz index 107
informed consent (IC) forms 27, 29, 32, 52, 82, 86; and consultation 63–64; doctor–patient relationships *45*; macrostructure 42–45
intentional/unintentional ableism 132
interactiveness 85
international nonproprietary name (INN) 34, 35

interpreters 15–18, 132, 134; ambiguous words 129; narrative perspective 141; strategies for 124–125
interpreting 15, 17, 19, 21–22, 124; accessibility and 69; channels 86; empathy and 119; telephone consultation and 64–65, 67
intertextuality (referential and functional) 18, 19
interviews 143, 144, 156, 159
intralingual translation 15, 69, 109, 110

Jakobson, R. 62
jargon 16, 41, 65, 72, 102
Jensen, M. N. 101, 102, 127

Khalikova, V. 25
Kialo 13

Lang, S. 127–128
language 6; CDA 140–141; corpus-based studies 139–140; fair and inclusive 131–134; non-verbal 23; oral communication 122–123; plain 128–129; social theory of 15; sociosemiotic theory of 61
lay audiences 91, *92*
learning difficulties, patients 72–73
legibility, concepts of 102
linguistic diversity 18
literacy 79, 108, 157

machine translation 160
Malinowski, B. 15
Mason, I. 19, 84
medical pluralism *see* pluralism
medical report 27, 32, 33; characteristics 49; macrostructure *48*; types 47
Medline 105
metonymy 16
mindfulness 9
mobile health technology 56, 57, 74
Mogami, S. 13
Montalt, V. 91
mother tongue 10, 14, 15, 90, 148, 149; audience 97
motivation 27, 90–91, 96
move (rhetorical) 103, 112
multiculturalism 106
multimodality 60; and accessibility 158–159; approach 61–62; good multimodal practice 65–67; informed consent 63–64; in medical consultation 62; oral and written in consultation 68; research process 158–159; roleplay 67–69; telephone consultation 64–65; visual and written resources 63
Munsour, E. E. 108

narrative analysis 141–142, 152, 154
neural mirror system 116
n-gram 139
non-verbal communication 23, 123

Olivia (fictional character) 27, 32–33, 82; communication problems 73, 101; face-to-face conversation 80; informed consent 116; patient-centred translation 101; PIL 32, 88; therapeutic process 62; visual and written resources 63
one-size-fits-all approach 74
onomatopoeias 58
oral communication skills, in empathy 119–125
original research articles (OAs) 38–40
Ortí, R. 22
Osler, W. 79

paralinguistic aspects, patients 23–24
parallel text 139
patient-centred communication 6–7; culture and context of situation 18–19; culture in 19–25; databases and social networks 162–163; definition 7; empathy in 117–119; patient-centredness 8–13; patient-centred translation 14–15; person-centred approach 7–8; references 161; research approaches, methods and tools in 138; research journals 162
patient-centred communication (PCC) 147
patient-centredness 8; core actions 9; DKA 11–12; empathy 9; factors 10; mindfulness 9; *vs.* patient-centricity 13; research process 148–149
patient-centred translation (PCT) 14–15; databases and social networks 162–163; domains *14*; references 161–162; research approaches, methods and tools in 138; research journals 162

patient-centricity 13
patient–doctor communication 60, 66, 120, 150
patient information leaflet (PIL) 16, *17*, 18, 27–29, 70, 88; sections of *34*
patient narratives 53; digital storytelling 54; illness 54; illness, experiences of 54–55; metaphorical expressions 54; translating/writing 56; web-based patient narratives 54
patient-reported outcomes 27, 51–52
patients: attitudes 96, 97; audience size 96; demographics 97; general categories of 94–95; health and illness 96; topic knowledge of 95–96; types of 92–94, *95*
patient summaries *see* summaries for patients (SPs)
Patient Voices 54–55
patronising language 91
Peñalver, A. 119
personality 10, 53, 82, 92, 108, 118, 163
person-centred approach 6–8
Pinazo, P. 124
pluralism 25, 106
power distance 22
pragmatic intentionality 59
Prieto-Velasco, J. A. 131
psychology 8, 20, 116, 117, 163
PsycINFO 163
PubMed 105, 163

readability, concepts of 102
readability formulas: comprehensibility 100, 106–109, **107**; patient-centred translation and communication 138–139
register 15, 18, 31, 82, 97
repertoires of genres 29
research 14, 102, 134–138; accessibility 158–159; artificial intelligence 160–161; audience analysis 156–157; CDA 140–141; comprehensibility 155–156; context 150–151; conversation analysis 145; corpus linguistics 139–140; culture 150–151; dramaturgical analysis 145–146; education 151–153; emotions 155–156; focus group 144; genres 153–154; interview 143; machine translation 160–161; multimodality 158–159; narrative analysis 141–142; patient-centredness 148–150; quantitative and numerical 108; readability formulas 138–139; resources for 161–163; survey 142–143; training 151–153; videoethnography 147
Riessman, C. K. 141
Rogers, C. R. 6–8
Roger's person-centred approach 8, *133*

Saiz-Hontangas, P. 131
Scopus 163
Semino, E. 54
Sidney School 18
Silverman, J. 66
situations *see* communicative situation
Skopos theory 79
Smith, S. G. 103
Smoke Free app 76
socioeconomic status 10, 103, 151
socio-professional cultures 20
summaries for patients (SPs) 27, 28, 33, 39–40; *Annals of Internal Medicine 40, 41*; translating/writing 42–43
surveys 33, 35, 142–143
Sustainable Development Goals 75
sympathy 116
synonymy 110, 129
systemic functional linguistics 15–16
Systems Knowledge Translation Center 36
Szigriszt Pazos, F. 107

telemedicine 56, 74, 76
telephone consultation 64–65, 87
tenor 18–19, 115; and personalising information 128
terminological density 49, 103
terminology 16, 38, 88, 106, 131; comprehensibility 112
text genre *see* genres
textual approaches 18–19

understanding, concepts of 16
US Food and Drug Administration 51

values 7, 10, 21, 33, 95, 141; cultural 9, 140; health and illness 24; individuals/groups of patients 6
videoethnography 147
video-reflexive ethnography (VRE) 147
visual and written resources, consultation 63

wearable technologies 76
web-based patient narratives 54
Web of Science 163
well-being 57, 90, 149; emotional 9, 87; and empowerment 14; mental 51; psychological 96
Williams, J. M. 161
World Health Organization (WHO) 35; blind and partially sighted patients 69; deaf and hard of hearing patients 71; e-health strategy 75; lack of comprehensibility 104; patient fact sheet *37*; poverty 75
written communication skills, in empathy 126–127; adjusting tenor 128; ambiguous words 129; credibility 130; empowering metaphors 130–131; fair and inclusive language 131–134; information 130; lexical choices 129; personalising information 128; small chunks and framing statements 129–130; specialised terms and plain language 128–129; strategies *132*; visual elements 131

Zethsen, K. K. 50, 91

FSC
www.fsc.org
MIX
Papier | Fördert
gute Waldnutzung
FSC® C083411

Kolibri 360 GmbH
Ferdinand-Jühlke-Straße 7
99095 Erfurt, Deutschland
produktsicherheit@kolibri360.de